THE CIMINELLI SOLUTION

THE CIMINELLI SOLUTION

A 7-Day Plan for Radiant Skin

SUSAN CIMINELLI

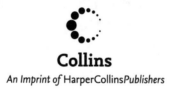

Collins
An Imprint of HarperCollinsPublishers

This book is written as a source of information only. The information contained in this book should by no means be considered a substitute for the advice, decisions or judgment of the reader's physician or other professional advisor.

All efforts have been made to ensure the accuracy of the information contained in this book as of the date published. The author and the publisher expressly disclaim responsibility for any adverse effects arising from the use or application of the information contained herein.

FIRST EDITION

Designed by rlf design

Printed on acid-free paper

Library of Congress Cataloging-in-Publication Data

Ciminelli, Susan.
    The Ciminelli solution : a 7-day plan for radiant skin / Susan Ciminelli.
        p.   cm.
    Includes index.
    ISBN-13: 978-0-06-077837-8
    ISBN-10: 0-06-077837-7
    1. Skin—Care and hygiene.   I. Title.

RL87.C48   2006
646.7'2—dc22   2005055121

06 07 08 09 10 DIX/RRD 9 8 7 6 5 4 3 2 1

To my wonderful mother and grandmother for all that they taught me throughout my life. Also to my dear and special father for his guidance, and my sweet and patient husband, Allan, for his unending support.

I am deeply grateful to Dr. Francesco Vettori and his beautiful wife, my cousin Andrea, who allowed me to live with them in Florence, Italy. Francesco was my first teacher in holistic healing, and his influence has helped shape my life forever. The warmth and comfort of their home, especially their kitchen, will stay with me for the rest of my days.

CONTENTS

ACKNOWLEDGMENTS

The contents of this book are based on thirty years of experience and practice in beauty, skin care, and wellness. Condensing this valuable information into a comprehensive book required a skilled team. I'd like to thank the following people for all that they have contributed to this project. To Coleen O'Shea, thank you for working with me to find the right home for this book and for overseeing its path. To Jodi Daley, thank you for your help early on in putting pen to paper. To Pamela Cannon, thank you for your organizing, writing, and editing skills. To Harriet Bell and the staff at William Morrow, thank you for all of your many efforts in producing this wonderful book.

THE CIMINELLI SOLUTION

Introduction

Beautiful skin and holistic health have both been incredibly important to me since I was a little girl growing up in Buffalo, New York. It was back then that I saw first-hand the connection between what was happening on my face and what was going on inside of my body. I was the second oldest of six children and extremely sensitive to what was going on around me. I loved the excitement of new babies in the house and wanted to help my mother as much as I could when she brought home a new little brother or sister. However, with a growing family comes growing stress, and I felt it every day.

Although I didn't understand the correlation then, that stress manifested as an imbalance in my system. Rashes would spring up, as well as little breakouts. Blemishes would appear every time I was constipated, which was often. What I know now is that the combination of family stress and processed "convenience" food, to which I found myself allergic, was the source of my problem. My body was showing me, through my skin, how *not* to eat and how *not* to live.

It's not as if the food in our family pantry was different from what was in many kitchen cupboards in the 1960s. The trend back then was toward convenience foods. Prepackaged and processed snacks and meals were time savers, but no one talked about how bad all the additives, artificial ingredients, white flour, sugar, fillers, and food coloring were for you. My body knew this, and it kept telling me that I wasn't getting what I needed in my diet. Lacking many of the essential vitamins, minerals, basic nutrients, and fiber my body was craving, the food seemed to be working against me rather than nourishing me.

By the time I was 15, I had been diagnosed with an ulcer, which the doctor said was the result of stress and my diet. I started to read everything I could on ancient forms of holistic healing including yoga and massage. While my friends would go to the mall and shop, I would sit on the floor of the local health food store and read books on nutrition, natural health, and healing, and magazines on food and exercise. On instinct, I started to practice yoga and perform shiatsu and reflexology on myself. My mother had always subscribed to the best and most sophisticated magazines, so I spent hours reading about exotic foods, discovering a whole new world of fresh ingredients and incredible combinations of foods that didn't come in a box. I began cooking in our kitchen, altering recipes, and trying new twists. Not so coincidentally, my skin problems began to fade.

I started practicing my newfound knowledge on friends. On weekends, I'd have my best friend stay over. From Friday night until Monday morning, I would feed her fruits, vegetables, and proteins, rather than the typical teenage diet of cola, pizza, and chips. Instead of watching TV, I'd give minifacials and steam open her pores over a pot of water infused with herbs such as rosemary and thyme. I'd whip up masks from pantry ingredients such as oatmeal and egg whites to draw out impurities, then I'd use a mixture of honey and pumpkin to smooth out her skin. By Monday morning, her complexion would be noticeably improved, and it wasn't long before she had clearer, more radiant skin. My research and instincts were paying off.

When I was 15, I moved to Italy for several months to stay with relatives. I shopped daily in the outdoor food markets, finding the freshest, most vibrant produce and delicacies, along with fragrant green olive oils. I watched as meals were prepared with little work and wonderful results. It was in Italy that I first discovered the satisfaction that comes from slowly eating small portions and the benefits of resting after meals. More important, I learned the value of good digestion and a settled stomach. My trip reinforced everything I'd already suspected about healthy living and good nutrition. When I returned to Buffalo, my ulcer was gone and my face was radiant.

Eager to apply all that I had learned about beauty throughout my teen years, my first job in the glamorous world of beauty was sweeping floors and giving shampoos in an upscale salon in Buffalo. As I'd shampoo the well-heeled ladies, I'd talk to them about their skin. And they'd listen. I'd make suggestions and they'd act on them. After I earned my cosmetology license, it wasn't long before my boss sent me to New York City to learn all about the latest equipment and most advanced skin care treatments.

When I first moved to New York City, I worked at Macy's selling an expensive French skin care treatment line. Eventually, I was transferred to Bloomingdale's, where I started doing facials in addition to selling the product line. My counter became a hub for potential customers who I would soon convert, as women would stop and eavesdrop while I spoke to other women about how to take care of their skin both externally and internally. A crowd would gather, and I would analyze one face, then the next. One woman who came by was going to a dermatologist once a week to have whiteheads removed. I told her to stop eating cow's milk dairy because I thought her body could not process the protein, fat, and/or additives in dairy products. Weeks later, she returned to the counter. The whiteheads were gone. And so were her weekly visits to the dermatologist.

Before long, I had developed a loyal clientele and decided it was time to begin treating them in a real spa environment. A legendary cosmetic giant had just built a state-of-the-art spa on the sixth floor of 601 Madison Avenue and hired me to work with her.

It was there that I furthered my knowledge of diet and how it affects the skin and the body. I often found that the women who ate fatty foods and cow's milk dairy had saddlebags, those large pouches of fat on the outside of the upper thighs. They also tended to have whiteheads that wouldn't go away. But as soon as they cut out the fat and dairy, their legs tended to slim down and their faces cleared up.

In 1983, after 3 years of solid spa experience and with only $300, I left to open my own business. Ironically, on my last day at the spa, I was giving a treatment to one of my clients who didn't know I was leaving, and she urged me to go out on my own because my methods were so much different from those of my old employer. I told her that I was leaving and she was thrilled. When she asked me what product line I was going to use, I told her that I was going to develop my own. This excited her even more.

When developing a line of skin care products, chemists often want to take the easy way out, sticking to tried-and-true methods. Every step of the way, I had to fight for each ingredient and every ratio. Although it's much easier to take a product that someone else has created and put a name on it, I insisted on developing my own and personally approving all of the ingredients and combinations. Moreover, I don't believe in animal testing. As a matter of fact, I was the "animal" for my product tests! Any product with my name on it had to be the most gentle and effective product possible. Over the years, I've added different products to my line but have always maintained the same standards using essential oils, seaweed extracts, and absolutely no harmful chemicals, mineral oil, or paraffin wax. These products that I have carefully developed and use at my spa are also available for use at home at www.susanciminelli.com.

By late 1983, I was running my own business from home, seeing clients such as Jerry Hall, Andie McDowell, Iman, and any number of other great beauties. I was mixing masks, brewing tea, preparing peels, and concocting crèmes in my kitchen. Somehow my clients never seemed to mind the informal surroundings. I earned the reputation of getting to the root of clients' problems very quickly, offering them all of my knowledge, intuition, and commitment to help them achieve beautiful skin.

At the same time, I started developing and creating holistic treatments to move energy through the body so that it could heal itself. It was also important for me to focus on nutrition because I saw that as the key to nourishing the skin. I had the beginning of my product line and had formed my own corporation. I had also become licensed in all types of massage. Until then, I hadn't really considered massage as an important part of my business plan, but when I started studying the body, I realized that the study of massage was really the study of not only muscles but also—and more important—the body's systems and how they all worked together. It was then that everything began to add up. Before I studied massage, most of what I *knew* about health and beauty came from intuition. But with this newfound knowledge, the relationship between the nervous system, the skeletal system, the connections between the meridians in the body, and the internal organs became clear. When I learned how connected the endocrine system was with the skin and the stomach, I finally had the facts, the hard-core basis for so much of what I'd intuitively known about the body. And I realized that so many doctors and Western health practitioners had overlooked how to teach people about these connections and how to use them to heal.

Once again, I found myself bucking the current skin treatment trends. During this time, it was all about *matte* skin. Basically, the thinking was that you had to dry the skin out so that it wouldn't break out. The method required you to wash with soap and hot water, then rinse with cold water. What I discovered, though, was that both hot and cold water will break the capillaries in your face. Hot water also makes you lose elasticity. I began telling my clients to wash with warm water and rinse with cool, which is much more gentle and protective of the skin. I also cautioned them against using soap, which dries out the skin and leaves a film. In fact, a gel cleanser was the first product I developed because of my aversion to soap. While everyone else was looking smooth and flat, my clients and I were looking dewy and fresh. Soon the country was choosing dewy and fresh. The trends were changing.

In 1990, I moved my business into the fashionable 601 Madison Avenue building where I had once worked for Helena Rubenstein. With a loving staff and a loyal clientele that now included Dustin Hoffman, Cindy Crawford, Al Pacino, Stephanie Seymour, and Sigourney Weaver, among others, I made sure that my new holistic state-of-the-art day spa retained the same warm and intimate atmosphere as I'd had in my own living room. The buzzword in skin care then was *cosmeceuticals,* which is loosely defined as the marriage of cosmetics and pharmaceuticals. Basically, dermatologists saw how popular good facialists and aestheticians were becoming with the public. In some cases, we were taking their clients away by offering natural healing and healthful alternatives to medicine. In reaction to this, the dermatologists started developing their own treatments to make women look younger. These treatments often consisted of burning, peeling, buffing, and basically destroying the precious skin they were attempting to help. My skin care program does just the opposite. It works from the inside out, helping women have healthier skin for a longer period of time.

Year after year, women buy into the hope that they'll have beautiful skin by using expensive creams, treatments, and elixirs, but it doesn't work that way. Even my natural and holistic product line can't prevent breakouts. Breakouts come from bad digestion, poor eating, and improper lifestyle choices. Good skin and good health don't come from one source. I'm 48 years old and have barely a wrinkle on my face, partly because I use natural products and mainly because I eat well, exercise, breathe properly, and take care of my skin.

A doctor can't do much with your skin if it's dried out, crinkled, and has no elasticity. He or she also can't help skin that has been bombarded by microdermabrasion, glycolic treatments, and silicone injections. Though we can't prevent aging, we can prevent *premature* aging by choosing to use products that will not destroy the skin and by eating a diet rich in healthy vegetable fats, lean proteins, vegetables, fruits, legumes, and whole grains.

Business was booming at 601 Madison, and I really thought I'd found a home for my clients and my staff. Then, after four years, we lost our lease and were forced out of our space with only three days' notice. We eventually moved to the ninth floor at the famed Bergdorf Goodman in Manhattan.

Today, the Susan Ciminelli Spa has a continually growing client list on both coasts, as well as in Europe, Asia, and the Middle East. Our products are distributed all over the world through the Internet, and I've had the pleasure of teaching on TV and numerous radio shows across the United States and in Great Britain and Japan. My clients are as diverse as I could ever hope for, from stay-at-home moms to doctors, presidents of corporations, and stars.

The last 30 years have taught me that good skin is not something we inherit. Rather, like so much in life, it's something we earn by making smart choices. Regardless of your age, skin type, and ethnic background, you can have good skin. *The Ciminelli Solution* provides you with the tools to make the right choices.

Each decision builds on itself, especially when it comes to your health and the health of your skin. If you abuse and neglect your muscles, they can't support you properly. If you eat poorly, it shows in brittle nails, limp and lifeless hair, and a body susceptible to bloating, cellulite, breakouts, pimples, premature wrinkles, and myriad diseases. Healthy skin comes from within. It is a result of what, when, and how you eat, and how well you take care of yourself—your body, your mind, and your spirit. A healthy body is the result of years of eating natural, organic foods rich in vitamins, minerals, and fiber; exercising regularly; breathing deeply; incorporating the tools needed to erase the effects of stress; and living positively day by day.

Many of my clients say they want to get rid of cellulite, rosacea, and saddlebags, but they refuse to give up the coffee and the sugar that I believe contribute to these conditions. One woman was anxious about the tight fit of her wedding dress and her blemished face, but she was reluctant to give up her daily large hot chocolate and whipped cream. I suggested switching to cleansing green tea because I thought she was bloated from the sugar in the hot chocolate, and her body and skin were reacting negatively to it. She took a chance, made that simple change, lost the inches, and looked beautiful in her wedding dress. Others wonder why their skin is red and broken out all the time, but when I suggest they stop using hot water on their face or cut down on spicy foods, which break capillaries, they balk. And it breaks my heart to see some of the unnatural chemical treatments such as glycolic acid, microdermabrasion, and acid peels being hyped as the way to a radiant complexion. The damage done by these treatments is not reversible. The answer is to live, eat, and buy *natural*. The rewards will be endless.

A beautiful complexion is like a flourishing garden. Success comes from nurturing your roots with the right food and activities. Long-lasting beauty is earned daily through diligence and care.

There isn't a quick-fix cream or fountain-of-youth fluid that will erase years of abuse; you need to make logical, healthy choices day to day, and each of these choices has obvious consequences. You'll sleep better, you'll have more energy, your moods will become more consistently elevated, and before you know it, you will see a whole new face looking back at you in the mirror.

Facing Your Face:
What's in the Mirror?

In order to take control of your skin, you must start by taking control of your overall health. Bad skin, blemishes, and breakouts tend to occur when your body is not in harmony. When your body is deprived of important nutrients, sleep, exercise, or relaxation, the result is an imbalance in your system. What you eat, how and when you eat it, if you exercise, if you choose to smoke, drink, or take drugs, and how well you breathe impact the quality of your skin. These choices are all paramount to balance and a healthy lifestyle. *The Ciminelli Solution* examines the causes of troubled skin and provides the tools and techniques to quickly and efficiently improve all skin types. Healthy skin is a by-product of a healthy body.

In order to achieve optimal health for your skin, you must understand the elements that can negatively impact it, including toxins, lifestyle, and the environment.

Toxins from the Outside In and the Inside Out

Toxins come in three forms: (1) those bombarding us from the environment around us, (2) those we create ourselves, and (3) those we put into our bodies. When it comes to environmental factors, ultraviolet (UV) rays, pollution, secondhand smoke, and radical changes in temperature break down the body's first line of defense: the skin. These are external factors that we can try to guard against, plan for, and to some extent avoid, but for the most part, they're out of our immediate control. The body generates toxins as it carries out its normal functions such as breathing and digestion. Those toxins we manufacture ourselves are the result of, among other things, stress, lack of sleep, and the effects of negative emotions on our bodies. The toxins that we ingest are often the simplest to avoid: cigarette smoke, alcohol, coffee, preservatives, refined sugar, hydrogenated oils, mercury from certain fish, antibiotics from farm-raised meat, and pesticides on fruits and vegetables. In order to avoid consuming toxins, try to exclude the following foods from your diet:

"Bad" Fats

Fat is necessary for your entire system to function properly, much like your car depends on oil to lubricate the engine. Your body functions the same way, requiring fat to lubricate its system and keep skin and hair hydrated. However, the types of fat you ingest can either help your body become a well-oiled machine or turn it into a clogged mess. That's why it's important to know the difference between good fats and bad fats.

There are four kinds of fats found in the food we eat: saturated, trans, monounsaturated, and polyunsaturated. The first two are considered "bad fats," while the second two are desirable.

Saturated fat is found in animal products, many dairy products, and tropical oils such as coconut and palm kernel oils. Popular diets such as the Atkins diet advocate eating a lot of cheese, meats, eggs, and other foods in this category, but the fact remains that too much animal or saturated fat is hard for the body to break down and can contribute to high cholesterol and heart disease. I have also found that your skin can get clogged as a result of eating too much of these foods.

Trans fat should be avoided at all costs. These fats are basically unsaturated or polyunsaturated fats that have been turned into saturated fats through a process called *hydrogenation,* wherein hydrogen molecules are added to good polyunsaturated oils such as soybean oil in order to make them solid or saturated fats. This new unhealthy fat is then added to processed and packaged foods such as chips, doughnuts, cookies, and a multitude of other snacks in order to extend their shelf life. According to the University of Maryland Medical Center, trans fats lower HDL (or good cholesterol) and increase LDL (or bad cholesterol) and, again, are much worse for you than the naturally saturated fats found in animal products.

Monosaturated and polyunsaturated fats, however, are the types you need in your system. The "good" fats found in olive oil, avocados, nuts, seeds, and fish such as salmon and sardines help attract moisture into the cells and keep skin lubricated—a must for beautiful skin.

If you are on a weight-loss program, do not completely eliminate good fats from your diet, or your skin will pay the price. This happened to my client, Gina, who was suffering from stress. Gina checked into a famous weight-loss clinic for 3 weeks. When she came back to see me, I was shocked by her appearance. She had lost weight and toned up, but she looked as if she had aged 10 years. She told me that the diet she had been on severely restricted fats. Her skin suffered permanent damage as a result, losing its elasticity and resulting in a dry, brittle, unattractive texture.

Healthy fats lubricate your body from the inside out. It is unhealthy to have a fat-free diet. Your skin and overall health will benefit from vegetable fats, fish oils, and nut and seed oils such as extra-virgin olive oil, salmon, mackerel, almonds, macadamia nuts, avocado, flaxseeds, and the other natural fats mentioned in the 7-Day Plan (see page 51) and the recipe section (see pages 95–193).

Refined Sugar

When I look at my clients' skin, I can tell immediately who consumes too much sugar. Sugar eaters tend to break out. They often have a blue-red cast to their skin similar to rosacea. Some suggest that with too much sugar in the system, the body's main source of fuel, blood glucose, accelerates the aging process via a chemical process called glycation. This is a process by which sugar crystals are broken down, causing caramelization. According to the *Journal of Investigative Dermatology,* glycation also results in the breakdown of dermal elastin and collagen, which exacerbates the skin's aging process and shows up as blotching, sagging, and wrinkling. Beyond that, sugar has been linked to the overproduction of insulin, which can lead to weight gain and diabetes.

Ironically, sugar is found in almost all foods. Look at the labels on processed foods. Notice how common one ingredient is—sugar. It may also go by the names of high-fructose corn syrup, corn syrup, maltose, and dextrose. I recommend to my clients that they be aware of the amounts and types of sugar they're eating. In chapter 4, you'll learn how to decipher food labels, but for now, just know how important it is to learn what's in the packaged food you're eating. Don't ever think that just because a product is found under the umbrella of "natural" that it is necessarily healthy. Be sure to read all labels and know how much sugar a product contains, even when shopping at a health food store.

If you are a sugar lover, there are a few things to help make life easier. Try using raw sugar instead of refined sugar, or substitute brown rice syrup, real maple syrup, date sugar, or honey for sugar, as I find they tend to break down more slowly in your system. But most important, stay away from processed foods and simple carbohydrates. Sometimes called simple sugars, simple carbohydrates include sucrose (table sugar), fructose (fruit sugar), and lactose (milk sugar). After the first few days of eliminating these harmful products and empty calories, your cravings will be curbed and you will start making healthier choices more easily.

Salt

Salt, or sodium, is a necessary part of your diet in that it retains the fluid in the body's cells and plasma, among other things. If you have too little sodium in your diet, you can become dehydrated, but too much can cause the body to retain fluid. This results in bloating, weight gain, and potential damage to the kidneys. According to the American Heart Association, we should consume only about 2½ grams of sodium a day, which amounts to about a teaspoon—a mere fraction of the sodium found in a serving of most of the processed and packaged foods we tend to eat every day. In fact, most Americans eat almost five times as much sodium as they should. Try to cut back on extra sodium by eliminating processed foods or adding it to your food at the table.

White Flour

White flour has been stripped of its vitamins and nutrients during processing. In its original form, the wheat kernel consists of three parts: (1) The outer layer is bran, which is high in B vitamins and minerals. Bran is also full of fiber, which helps digestion and the elimination of toxins from the system. (2) The center part is wheat germ, which contains vitamin E and essential fatty acids. (3) What's left over is the endosperm, which is basically starch that is bleached using chemicals such as aluminum chloride, chlorine, and calcium sulfate, none of which help promote a healthy body. Unfortunately, white or "enriched" flour is the basis for too many staples in the American diet and shows up in most commercially packaged breads, baked goods, and pastas.

Preservatives and Other Packaged Food Ingredients

Preservatives, additives, dyes, and artificial sweeteners are next on the list of things to avoid. Many chemicals added to food to preserve freshness or add flavor can negatively affect the skin. A diet loaded with additives can contribute to skin problems such as eczema, adult acne, dry patches, rosacea, loss of elasticity, and premature aging.

Sodium Nitrite

Sodium nitrite is a chemical that is used as a preservative and color fixative in many processed meats such as hot dogs and bologna to keep them looking "fresh." The textile industry uses sodium nitrite in dyes and bleaches as well as in metal coatings for phosphatizing and detinning. Considering all this, is it really something you want to put into your body? My rule of thumb is if it isn't fresh naturally, don't eat it.

Alcohol

We all know drinking too much alcohol is not good for you. Not only does it negatively impact the liver over a prolonged period, but it also dehydrates the skin. If you are inclined to consume alcohol, I suggest drinking a glass of wine rather than hard liquor or beer. Wine has less alcohol per volume, and I have found it to be gentler on the system and less dehydrating.

If you are inclined to overdo it every now and then, here are a few hints to avoid dehydrating your skin, or to rehydrate and recover from alcohol consumption: Drink one glass of spring water after each alcoholic drink. This will dilute the amount of alcohol coming into your system as well as help keep your body hydrated. Drink 8 ounces of water combined with the juice from one-half lemon the morning after drinking to hydrate and cleanse the body. Also try to eat sliced cucumbers and fruits high in water content such as watermelon, cantaloupe, and honeydew melon throughout the day. When the colon is dehydrated, it cannot properly eliminate toxins from your system, thus creating an imbalance that can lead to blemishes on your face, dark circles under your eyes, and lack of energy in your body.

Improper Nutrition and Digestion

A diet that contains junk food is high in calories and refined carbohydrates such as white flour and white sugar, and it is low in vitamins, minerals, and phytonutrients, which are the natural substances found in fruits, vegetables, and whole grains that benefit health and beauty and reduce the risk of disease. A nutrient-deficient diet does not give the skin what it needs to look its best. It's not just coincidental that the people I've heard complain about the dark circles under their eyes, cellulite, pimples, constipation, and a host of other physical problems are the ones who indulge in soda, junk food, and fast food on a regular basis.

Take a look at your own day-to-day food intake. The typical American diet includes too much meat, white flour, sugar, artificial sweeteners, coffee, and soda. All of these affect your body by causing an imbalance in the pH level, the degree of acidity or alkalinity. The body functions best when acidity and alkalinity are in balance. The wrong diet can exacerbate everything from blemishes on your skin to more serious diseases.

Along with what you eat, when and how you eat affects the skin, too. For example, meals eaten after 8:00 P.M. may not be adequately digested and may turn into toxic waste in the stomach and intestines, which can cause recurring breakouts, cellulite, constipation, and weight gain. It is important to eat slowly and chew adequately for proper digestion, and some experts suggest not drinking too much liquid with meals, as this will dilute the enzymes needed for efficient digestion. When the body is not digesting efficiently, toxins build up and wreak havoc on the skin.

According to Indian meditation masters and the principles of Ayurveda (one of the oldest forms of medicine in the world), the golden rule for proper digestion is one-third air, one-third food, and one-third liquid in your stomach at any given meal. In keeping with this, I encourage you to eat a number of small meals throughout the day rather than only one or two large meals. Eating until you are full may leave you uncomfortable and unable to properly digest the food you have just consumed. Eating small meals to keep yourself satiated helps maintain a consistent ratio of air to food to liquid, which will lend itself to more optimal health. By following this golden rule, digestion, absorption, and ultimately elimination will be more efficient. We will talk more about this golden rule in chapter 4.

"Dis-ease" Creates Disease

When toxins build up in your system and don't exit properly, your body tends to show the effects of this buildup in numerous ways. Long before serious illness manifests itself, internal and external factors affect the body, causing what I refer to as "dis-ease," or lack of energy flow. These factors include poor nutrition, environmental conditions, stress, heredity, and lack of proper sleep and exercise. Dis-ease is the first indicator that the body is out of balance.

When my client, Rachael, came to me for a facial, she had a horrible rash around her nose and nostrils that her dermatologist had diagnosed as "a cross between eczema and acne." The antibiotics she took for weeks did nothing for her. I suggested that she increase her daily water intake. In addition, I recommended that each day she should drink one 8-ounce glass of spring water with one tablespoon of black cherry juice concentrate. In less than a week, the rash that had been plaguing her for more than 3 months was gone. The black cherry juice acted as a natural antiinflammatory, and the water helped flush her system of toxins more quickly and efficiently. In this case, the dis-ease was addressed before it became more serious.

Signs of dis-ease reveal themselves with symptoms that we often feel are not serious enough to investigate. The immune system, which is equipped to neutralize and eliminate toxins, may not be acutely out of equilibrium, but it is working overtime to compensate for irregularities. So are certain organs, including the organs of filtering and purification (i.e., the liver and kidneys) and the organs of elimination (i.e., the lungs, large intestine, bladder, and skin).

The *liver* is the body's major purification organ. It absorbs nutrients from food and removes harmful waste from the body, among other functions. The *kidneys* sift out waste and extra water from the breakdown of tissues and from food and also regulate the amount of water in the body. The *lungs* eliminate toxins through gaseous waste (carbon dioxide), the *large intestine* through solid waste, the *bladder* through liquid waste, and finally toxins exit the skin in the form of perspiration and breakouts through tiny pores and sweat glands. The *colon* is the part of the digestive system that moves waste from the *small intestine* to the rectum (the small intestine is where carbohydrates are digested). As the colon transports this waste, it absorbs water and toxins. When the colon is backed up, the other eliminative organs, including the skin, get congested as well.

The *lymphatic system* is important to the body's detoxification efforts as well. It is a network of fluid, glands, organs, and vessels that move waste and nutrients that are too large to pass through the circulatory system, which only carries blood. The lymphatic system carries lymph, a clear fluid in which cells bathe. Lymph moves through lymph vessels and passes through lymph nodes, which act as purification centers. When lymph vessels and nodes become stagnant, they become clogged with debris and toxic waste. This can negatively impact the immune system. A sedentary lifestyle can create poor circulation, which may allow toxins to accumulate, causing cells to function improperly. Each organ has its job to do; if even one is imbalanced, overtaxed, or overtoxicated, the entire system is thrown off and the immune system is impaired, much like a domino effect.

Our bodies are constantly giving us signals of dis-ease: headaches, menstrual cramps, monthly breakouts, feelings of lethargy and sluggishness, sleeplessness. Even a funny taste in your mouth is an indicator that something is not working correctly. Long before Western medicine may determine that something is going wrong, the symptoms of dis-ease are already giving off warning signals. Our job is to pay attention to these signals and do something about them before minor issues become major problems.

Learning how to listen to your body is the key. Yoga, meditation, relaxation techniques, and calm breathing all help keep energy flowing freely as well as keep you in tune with the constant signals of possible dis-ease. These healthful practices are covered in the chapters ahead. Massage, reflexology, and acupuncture are also highly beneficial for stress reduction.

It's important to focus your body's energy. My client, Elizabeth, was really out of sorts. Her meeting with a new client had not gone well and she had missed a parent–teacher conference at her son's school. When she got home, she started to cook dinner and cut her finger while slicing onions. A little later, as she was removing a pot from the stove, she burned her hand. Finally, while serving dinner, she dropped a carton of milk on the floor. When she told me about this, she said that when the milk spilled, she just stared at it and realized all the things that had happened were a result of not being focused. Elizabeth had disconnected with what she was doing and left herself vulnerable to mishaps.

Focus your energy on living a healthy lifestyle. The more disconnected you are with your body, the more likely you are to miss the signals it gives you every day. Dis-ease is a signal and a blessing. In my 25 years of working on thousands of people from all walks of life, I have observed that dis-ease almost always shows up on the face.

The bottom line is that our bodies talk to us. As we age, the conversation changes. We must learn how to read and listen to this ongoing dialogue.

Free Radicals: Targeting the Enemy

Sun, pollution, toxic foods, chemicals, cigarette smoke, stress, lack of sleep, and lethargic lifestyles all have one thing in common: they create the single most detrimental aging agent, free radicals. In order to understand what free radicals do, we need to know how they are formed. As you know, the body is made up of billions of cells, and cells are made up of molecules. Molecules are made up of atoms, and atoms are made up of protons, neutrons, and electrons, all swimming around the nucleus or center of the atom and binding together with other atoms through the electrons. When the bond between two atoms is weak and the atoms split, forcing one atom to steal the other one's electron, free radicals are formed. In essence, a free radical tries to get back the lost electron and, in doing so, attacks anything in its way. This disturbs the balance in the atoms and the molecules and eventually weakens and kills the cell, cell structures, and even the genetic material within the cell. If left unchecked, free radicals can destroy skin and internal tissue and even contribute to major diseases such as cancer and heart disease.

Antioxidants prevent free radicals from spreading and damaging your cells by adding the missing electron and stopping the chain reaction of destruction. Keeping your skin healthy, fresh, and young starts at the cellular level. Where free radicals thrive, skin sags, blotches, wrinkles, and loses elasticity. Therefore, one of the best things you can do for your skin is eat a diet rich in fruits and vegetables, which are loaded with antioxidants.

Elements and the Environment: The Role They Play on Your Skin

As you know, the sun is one of your skin's worst enemies. The atmosphere above us has been changing because of holes in the ozone layer. The sun is stronger, the rays more penetrating. And that "healthy tan" we all wanted as kids is now a dangerous precursor to skin cancer as well as an invitation to wrinkles, sunspots, and loss of elasticity.

Maria is one of my favorite clients at my Montecito practice. A mother of three, she takes care of herself with proper nutrition, exercise, and yoga. She has also spent too much time in the California sun. The first time I gave her a facial, her skin felt very dry and brittle and looked flaky. She told me her main goal was for her skin to look younger, but she made it clear that she had no intention of giving up her sunbathing. I told her that without giving up the sun, there was little anyone could do for her skin. Although my products did give her a beautiful glow and people noticed the difference in her skin right away, I knew that no product in the world would reverse the sun damage.

Several months after we met, Maria and her family traveled to the south of France for a vacation, and she noticed how incredibly sun-damaged and old-looking the people on the beach were. Their entire bodies were completely wrinkled, and they looked awful. It was then that Maria decided to be more careful about the sun. On went the sunscreen and up went the umbrella. Today, by taking the proper steps to prevent further skin damage, Maria has a more radiant complexion. Her skin has regained elasticity, become more dewy and supple, and she looks ten years younger in spite of some irreversible skin damage. Limiting sun exposure is still the best way to have healthy-looking skin with a combination of diet, exercise, and healthy lifestyle practices.

Listening to Your Skin's Messages

Skin is the body's largest and most diverse vital organ. It breathes, regenerates, rids the body of toxins, and protects muscles, bones, joints, and vital organs. It also takes an environmental beating every single day. It's important to treat your skin with the same kind of care and respect you would treat any other major organ. For example, if you knew certain spicy foods hurt your stomach, you'd stay away from them. You need to pay the same care and attention to your skin.

If the products in your skin care routine contain acids, alcohol, mineral oils, or paraffin, then you are prematurely aging your skin. If you're a smoker, heavy drinker, overstressed, or live in a heavily polluted environment, your skin and your health are paying the price.

Breaking out means that your skin is eliminating toxins. Don't ignore it. You wouldn't ignore a lump, a cough, or a pain in your chest, so don't ignore irritations on your skin. They are signals that there is an imbalance in your body. Often, there is a direct correlation between where the breakout occurs and the part of your body that is sending the signal.

If you break out a quarter-inch from the sides of your nose, just before the apple of your cheeks, this may reflect what's going on in your stomach. The types, amount, and condition of the food you eat can have a huge effect on your stomach. For instance, too much food jammed into the stomach makes it hard for it to function. Picture your washing machine packed so full that it becomes overloaded and imbalanced. There's no way your clothes are going to get clean, and with the washer that full, you're probably looking at a messy overflow onto the laundry room floor as well. Your stomach works in much the same way.

Weak or sensitive stomachs are overworked and abused stomachs. If you're constantly eating the wrong foods, not chewing thoroughly, eating too quickly, or eating late at night, you're asking for trouble. The drug industry has made billions of dollars treating stomach conditions such as acid reflux disease, ulcers, acid indigestion, and a multitude of other ailments. Ironically, most of these conditions can be attributed to poor eating habits and can often be alleviated with a change in diet.

Eat when you're calm. If you are in an agitated state, it will hinder digestion. If you're not calm at mealtime, take deep, slow breaths for about 5 minutes to allow yourself to relax. Eat your last meal before 8:00 P.M. Take small bites, chew thoroughly, and eat slowly. Remember to take time to breathe in between bites. These things may all sound simple, but if you're breaking out in the area alongside the nose, you're probably not doing one or more of them on a regular basis.

Breaking out on the forehead may be a direct reflection of what's going on in your small intestine. If you eat on the run or while you're anxious or agitated, you may not chew your food thoroughly. This gives rise to a domino effect of problems, whereby food isn't broken down properly in your stomach and small intestine, which results in poor assimilation of nutrients into your system and problems in elimination, leading to constipation. So relax. Slow down. Breathe deeply. You wouldn't rush through a workout and risk damaging muscles and bone. Likewise, don't rush through meals. Don't shove as much food as will fit into your mouth. Try and chew each bite a minimum of 20 times. It will slow down the eating process and help you digest your food properly.

If you're wondering if your fatty food intake matters, look into your eyes. A yellowing of the whites of your eyes and breaking out between your eyebrows is a reflection of stressing the liver. The liver is a factory, producing substances such as bile, which helps break down and digest fats and cholesterol in order to maintain and balance bodily functions. The liver performs a huge juggling act, excreting and eliminating waste products, especially those in the medications and chemicals we consume every day. It also stores vitamins, filters poisons, and synthesizes proteins. When you tax it with fatty foods, it has to work overtime. Breaking out between your eyes is your liver's first signal that it needs a rest from the toxins you're consuming on a daily basis. Besides balancing your diet and cutting out as many prepackaged and nonorganic foods as possible, one easy thing you can do to help cleanse your system is to drink a large glass of spring water mixed with 1 tablespoon of organic apple cider vinegar or the juice of one-half lemon every day. Also, eat lots of dark leafy vegetables for the beneficial nutrients they contain.

I have found that breaking out on the temples is a reflection of what's going on in the gallbladder. The gallbladder is right behind the liver. Its job is to store and release the bile produced by the liver. While we eat, the gallbladder contracts, releasing bile into the small intestine. Too many fatty foods result in an imbalance in the gallbladder.

If you break out on your chin, it's usually indicative of a problem in your endocrine system. Think of your endocrine system as your body's transport system for hormones. The endocrine system is made up of the pituitary, thyroid, adrenal, salivary, and sweat glands. It produces hormones and carries them throughout the system. Most meat, unless it is organic, contains hormones and antibiotics. Too much in your diet may throw off your endocrine system by creating a turf war between your hormones and the ones introduced into your system through meat and dairy. Limiting your meat intake and eating organic foods can be incredibly beneficial to the endocrine system.

Clogged pores may be a sign that your system is being burdened by waste trapped in your colon. Waste enters the colon in mostly liquid form. The colon then absorbs any excess water, electrolytes, and vitamins. By the time the remaining waste passes through the colon, it is released as solid waste. If the colon is blocked and waste remains there, autointoxication results, whereby the toxins and parasites from this waste are absorbed into your bloodstream and cause a multitude of serious diseases, eventually breaking down your immune system. Drinking ample amounts of water, as well as eating fresh fruits, leafy greens, and other fibrous foods, helps keep things moving through your colon.

The good news is whether it comes to dis-ease or imbalances that lead to breakouts, there is a way to help your body eliminate the internal and external poisons that threaten it and your skin. It is called detoxification. Chapter 2 will provide you with the tools, techniques, and treatments to detoxify your body for better skin and better overall health and vitality.

TWO

Tools, Treatments, and Techniques for Beautiful Skin

Once you know what your health challenges are, you can do something about them. Detoxification is the cleansing of the internal organs to restore your body and your skin to a healthy condition. If properly used, detoxification techniques can strengthen the organs of elimination and help the body purge itself of toxins. I can't stress to you enough how interconnected rebalancing your skin is with rebalancing your life. It is a process of nurturing the self physically, emotionally, and mentally not only through smart food choices but through activities such as yoga, meditation, exercise, and time management as well as skin care and different forms of massage. This chapter will provide you with the information to help make this process easier, more fun, and above all, effective.

The Basics of Detoxification

There are several ways to detoxify the body and the skin. Diet and exercise are the cornerstones. A diet of fresh fruits, fresh herbs and vegetables, and whole grains gives the body the nutrients it needs to cleanse and eliminate poisons stored in the colon. These foods are packed with vital nutrients, water, and fiber that not only nourish the body but also help the colon and kidneys eliminate toxins through bowel movements and urine. Aerobic exercise increases the metabolism and gets your body up and running. As you burn calories through activities such as walking, running, and swimming, your body heats up and circulation is improved. This moves the blood through the kidneys faster and expedites the natural cleansing process when liquid waste is eliminated through the bladder. Perspiration gets rid of toxins through your skin, and when your breathing is heavier, toxins are expelled more quickly from your lungs. Weight training is the key to strengthening muscles, bones, and joints, keeping the body strong and healthy from the inside out. It protects bone mass from the effects of age as well as eliminates toxic residues and stagnant biochemicals from the muscular system.

You may have heard that fasting—drinking only water or fresh fruit or vegetable juices—is a good way to detoxify. It can be, but the problem is it can also be a real shock to the system. While fresh juices do supply a substantial number of nutrients, they don't offer enough by themselves. In addition, fasts that consist only of water can backfire, depleting the body of the nutrients it needs to cleanse itself, such as antioxidants, vitamins, protein (the liver needs it to do its detoxification work), and fiber. I prefer that my clients change their diets, incorporating healthy fruits, vegetables, good fats, and lean protein. My 7-Day Plan (see pages 51–94) helps to jump-start this healthy eating program.

When you stop overloading your body with toxins, the organs of elimination have the time and energy to work more effectively. Cleansing the colon is particularly important because it must be clear before it can accept waste from other organs and then eliminate. To help this process along, I advise my clients to eat plenty of fiber, drink water with lemon for cleansing, and eliminate cow's milk dairy products, as some research has shown that these dairy products are more difficult for some people to digest and absorb. If clients still want to eat dairy on occasion, I recommend that they include radishes or daikon (Japanese radish) in the same meal as the dairy. I have found these root vegetables to help in the digestion of animal proteins and animal fats.

Laura came to me with extensive whiteheads on her cheeks. She had combination skin and tried to treat her whiteheads with soap, water, and alcohol-based toners, believing this cleaning method would get rid of what she thought was an external problem on her face. Yet all this did was irritate her skin, dry it out, and cause premature aging. Some facialists and dermatologists would have removed the whiteheads, dried out the skin with acids and harsh peels, and considered the problem handled, but when Laura came to me for a facial, I changed her cleansing routine from a drying soap to a gel cleanser and an algae-based gentle peel.

When I asked Laura about her diet, she told me that because she was over 40, she thought she needed more calcium to help prevent osteoporosis, so she'd started eating more dairy and taking a calcium supplement. I suggested eating more calcium-rich but dairy-free foods such as broccoli, kale, chickpeas, salmon, sardines, and tofu. Laura was reluctant to eliminate dairy completely from her diet, so I suggested that she substitute active Greek yogurt, with the added benefit of acidophilus, a healthy bacteria that helps the colon break down food, for cottage cheese. Instead of Brie, I suggested goat cheese, since I have found it easier to digest. I also suggested that she snack on celery and radishes and have fresh lemon juice in at least one glass of water a day. I was confident that consuming less cow's milk dairy would help the whiteheads go away. She called me the next week to report that she went right out after her facial and bought some radishes, celery, and lemons, which she started consuming immediately, cut down on her dairy, and the whiteheads were rapidly disappearing. Laura didn't drastically change her eating, nor did she deprive herself of anything she liked. She just made a few adjustments that helped her skin from the inside out.

The more you know about what's in the foods you eat, the healthier your choices will be. While it's important to eliminate processed foods, nonorganic meats, white sugar, white flour, coffee, and soda from your diet, I also recommend saying good-bye to foods fried in butter, lard, or hydrogenated, partially hydrogenated, or other unhealthy fats. Stick to the good fats such as extra-virgin olive oil, raw nuts, seeds, and avocados to get and stay healthy. Including good fats lubricates the body and the skin. This is essential not only for optimal health but also for a radiant complexion.

I have found that one of the primary benefits of detoxification is the rebalancing of the body's acid-alkaline state. As your body detoxifies or cleanses itself, it rebalances itself as well. Most people's bodies are overly acidic, primarily from a day-to-day diet that includes too many animal products such as meat, cow's milk dairy, white flour, sugar, artificial sweeteners, coffee, and soda. Signs that your blood is too acidic include skin eruptions, sugar cravings, lethargy, headaches, mood swings, obesity, cramps, and heavy periods. Acidity also causes bacteria to grow in the body, which then shows up on the skin through breakouts and discoloration such as a blue-red cast.

To achieve optimum health and well-being, the body's chemistry needs to be in balance. Leafy green vegetables, fruits, certain grains such as millet, and wild and brown rice are rich in alkaline salts such as potassium chloride, calcium sulfate, and calcium fluoride that help lower acidity in your body: the alkaline salts act as acid binders to move the acid waste out of fluids in your system while the fiber keeps things flowing. More information on these important grains is in chapter 4.

Tools for Detoxification

Incorporating the following changes into your daily routine will result in your skin's transformation from dull or lackluster to radiant. My 7-Day Plan (see page 51) puts each of these principles into practice. My hope is that you will eventually incorporate them into your lifestyle for a lifetime of beauty and health.

Foods from the Earth

There's a reason your mother told you to eat your fruits and vegetables—they're excellent sources of fiber, and they're rich in vitamins, minerals, antioxidants, and phytochemicals, all nutrients your body and skin need to stay healthy.

One good rule of thumb: choose organic produce whenever possible. Organic refers to the way foods—including fruits and vegetables, grains, and meat—are grown, raised, and/or processed. Organic foods are farmed without the use of toxic pesticides and fertilizers, and they are minimally processed without artificial ingredients, preservatives, and other chemicals. Organic meat, poultry, eggs, and dairy products come from animals that are not given growth hormones or antibiotics. When you support your local organic community, you can feel good knowing that you are helping to protect your internal environment as well as Mother Earth. Fortunately, organically grown produce, meats, and poultry are becoming more readily available across the United States. However, if you can't find a source that's convenient for you, check on-line (see Sources), as there is a strong on-line community of producers that will ship virtually anywhere.

If for some reason you're unable to buy organic products, you can still reduce your intake of toxic chemicals by washing and peeling conventionally grown fruits and vegetables. Use either a store-bought fruit and vegetable wash (see Sources) or a diluted mixture of one-quarter teaspoon eco-friendly liquid dish detergent to one sinkful of water. Scrub the fruits and vegetables gently in cold water and rinse them completely. Also, eating a wide variety of produce helps to minimize your exposure to pesticides that are used exclusively on individual crops.

No single fruit or vegetable provides all of the nutrients you need for optimal health. The key lies in eating a variety of them. The simplest way to do this is to buy and eat produce that is in season and, if possible, locally and organically grown. If you live in Connecticut, it's better to wait until early summer to savor strawberries rather than buy the ones from California in January. While produce that is in season depends on where you live, in general, opt for fresh vegetables, greens, and herbs whenever possible. In the summer, the body thrives on fruits and vegetables that contain a large amount of water such as melons and peaches. In the fall, apples, grapes, and squash are good choices. In the winter, root vegetables such as turnips, parsnips, carrots, and sweet potatoes are high in minerals and help fortify the immune system for cold and flu season. And, to guarantee you're getting all the vitamins and minerals you need, make sure you're eating both vegetables grown above the ground and root vegetables grown below the ground, such as turnips, parsnips, rutabagas, beets, onions, and carrots.

Water: The Essential Element

Water is one of the most important elements of the human body, making up approximately 70 percent of our muscle and about 75 percent of our brain. It is an essential part of a healthy diet and plays a vital role in the proper functioning of the body. Water is also an essential factor for beautiful skin. It is not just that adequate water

⚜ EATING FOR DETOXIFICATION ⚜

As you focus on eating for better health and better skin, here are some suggestions:

- Eliminate processed foods.

- Limit or eliminate full-fat dairy products and fatty meats.

- Always opt for sautéing foods in olive oil.

- Do not drink soda.

- Eat slowly and chew thoroughly for proper digestion.

- Never eat when you are agitated.

- Spend 5 minutes deep breathing before you begin each meal.

- Don't eat after 8:00 P.M.

- Eat small meals throughout the day rather than large meals.

- Eat locally grown organic food that is in season whenever possible.

- To guarantee you're getting all the vitamins and minerals you need, make sure you're eating both vegetables grown above the ground and below the ground.

- Every day drink at least one-half ounce of spring water per pound that you weigh. If you weigh 130 pounds, then you should drink approximately 8 glasses of spring water each day.

- Start your day with a Detoxification Beverage (pages 49–50).

intake helps the skin stay smooth, soft, and glowing, but more important, it is necessary if your body is going to efficiently eliminate toxins, both natural and man-made. Toxins trapped in your body affect not only your health and well-being but the quality of your skin as well. If there is one single thing you do to improve your health and skin care, it should be drinking more water.

Eliminating the danger of dehydration is another primary reason to incorporate plenty of water into your diet. In fact, you should never wait until you are thirsty to drink water, since thirst is actually one of the last signs of dehydration. In essence, by the time you feel thirsty, your body is already in a state of dehydration. Drinking bottled spring water (not just liquids) throughout the day is the only way to keep the water balance in your body. This, in turn, helps keep all of your systems running smoothly, including your skin. If I don't drink at least 3 liters of water each day, I don't feel as healthy as I normally do, nor does my skin look as smooth and clear. Yes, I am always in and out of the bathroom, but I'm much healthier and look years younger than most people my age. I advise my clients to drink one-half ounce of water for every pound they weigh. So, for example, if you weigh 150 pounds, then you should drink 75 ounces of spring water, or roughly 8 to 10 glasses every day.

Deep Breathing

Next to eating right, breathing correctly is one of the best ways to keep the body running efficiently on several levels. On a physical level, proper breathing keeps the blood oxygenated, the mind and body relaxed, and the digestive tract functioning in a nonagitated state. On a deeper level, breathing is essential to psychological and emotional health. Breathing focuses the body and the mind, moving them into a rhythm that eases stress, lightens the spirit, and ultimately relaxes the body so that it can function properly.

Eastern methods of healing and wellness have incorporated breathing exercises into their regimens for thousands of years, but only recently has Western medicine acknowledged their potential. When you are detoxing, deep breathing exercises and yoga poses (see chapter 6) are essential for stimulating all of the right organs, for proper elimination, natural lymphatic drainage, and overall rebalancing. It is especially important to practice deep breathing just before you turn in for the night. You will no doubt go to sleep calmer and achieve a more restful night's sleep.

Yoga

Yoga is a six-thousand-year-old practice that combines a series of poses called asanas, breathing exercises, and meditation to increase the body's health and physical, mental, and spiritual well-being. Yoga was conceived in India and made its way westward over the last century to become the cornerstone of holistic health. Its benefits have even been touted by such mainstream organizations as the American Heart Association and Yale University School of Medicine. Yoga can be credited with increasing energy and reducing blood pressure and body fat, but it is also valued for moving the body and the mind into a healthier, more relaxed state. Yoga opens up energy channels, which may help take you from a state of dis-ease to a state of free energy flow.

Aerobic Exercise

Speed walking, swimming, cycling, trampoline jumping, or other gentle aerobic exercise helps improve circulation and metabolism. As little as 30 minutes four times a week can make a huge difference in your body's efficiency. I recommend speed walking as an optimal exercise for my 7-Day Plan. While speed walking, try to achieve a pace of 1 mile every 12 to 15 minutes, or 4 to 5 miles per hour. Drink plenty of spring water while you are walking. If possible, walk on a slight incline. (Be careful about the incline if you have lower back or knee problems.) If you are walking on a treadmill, set the incline no higher than 3 to start and gradually progress to 5. Too much of an incline may cause discomfort and stress to your lower back. If you regularly participate in other aerobic activity such as tennis, cycling, swimming, or dancing, substitute that for speed walking.

Try a number of different exercises and stick with what you enjoy most, whether it's going to a gym a few times a week, walking to and from work, or riding your bike around town. All of these forms of exercise will help benefit the cardiovascular and circulatory systems.

Teeth and Tongue Brushing

Potentially harmful bacteria grows in your mouth throughout the day. In order to prevent this bacteria from contaminating the food you ingest and traveling into your digestive system, you should brush your teeth and your tongue at least three times a day, preferably before each meal. To clean your teeth, gently brush them with a soft toothbrush. Use a tongue cleaner (available at pharmacies and natural food stores) to gently scrape your tongue clean. Finally, several times a week, rinse your mouth with 1 teaspoon of hydrogen peroxide added to 8 ounces of water—a natural detoxifier.

Abdominal Massage

You can encourage elimination of solid toxins through the colon by performing a gentle abdominal massage in the morning when you wake up or right before you go to bed at night. Lie on your back with your knees bent. Place a few pillows under your knees to help support your lower back. Roll a small hand towel lengthwise (about 3 inches in diameter) and place it under the nape of your neck for support. Place 1 tablespoon of castor oil (a powerful oil that helps the body purge its waste and promotes circulation in the area on which it is being used) on your abdomen and massage clockwise in slow, deep methodical strokes. Think of your abdominal area as the face of a clock where 12:00 is right under your sternum, or chest bone. One o'clock is to the left, and so on. The strokes should be strong and purposeful but loving. After about 20 strokes, place a thick cotton towel over your abdomen for about 15 minutes (or overnight, if you prefer). Remember to breathe deeply and slowly to relax your nervous system. This whole process should only take about 20 minutes.

The combination of abdominal massage, Smooth Move Tea blend (see page 230), drinking more water, and eating more healthfully will result in more efficient elimination. This helps clear up breakouts, reduces darkness and puffiness under the eyes, and strengthens your immune system because you are efficiently eliminating toxic waste from your system.

Skin Care Treatments

As you know by now, the appearance of your skin reflects the food choices you make, how well you digest and assimilate that food, and how efficiently you eliminate the waste. Remember that even a meal made up of the healthiest food choices can remain undigested if you're eating on the run, drinking too much liquid at the same time, are agitated while you eat, or eat too late at night. This undigested food results in excessive fat and waste, which makes its presence known on your face in the form of pimples and breakouts. The way you care for your skin on a daily basis is just as important. The toxins that accumulate in your system manifest themselves in the form of breakouts, redness, cysts, poor elasticity, and dryness. By adhering to a good skin care regimen and following some basic rules, you can help your body and skin to detoxify and look healthy.

Proper Cleansing and Moisturizing

The first rule is the simplest: Wash your hands frequently and thoroughly. Always make sure that anything touching your face is clean, starting with your hands. Buy a dozen or so inexpensive washcloths and towels to keep on hand, and use a clean washcloth and clean towel every time you wash your face. This simple precaution will minimize the chance of spreading bacteria from a used towel onto your face. Furthermore, try to use white towels so that when you launder them you can use a bit of bleach or "green" antibacterial detergent to help kill residual bacteria.

The most important skin care rule concerns soap. Never use it on your face or body. Soap is harsh and always leaves a film that suffocates the surface of the skin, stripping it of its natural hydration and leaving it flaky and dull. Since this film cannot be rinsed off, it causes your pores to stretch, dries out your skin, and causes it to itch, especially in winter. Instead, always use a gel cleanser, which cleans deeper than soap and leaves no residue. It should be gentle enough for a baby's skin and should not contain detergents or chemicals, but it should be effective in removing light makeup.

The best way to cleanse is to wash with warm water and rinse with cool water. Using water that is too hot or too cold can damage your capillaries and cause your skin to sag. Unfortunately, once your capillaries actually break, there is nothing that can be done to reverse this damage.

I live in New York City, where the air is fouled with car exhaust and scores of other toxins, so I wash my face twice in the morning and twice at night to ensure that I am getting my skin superclean. It's similar to the "rinse, lather, repeat" directions you find on the back of a shampoo bottle. The first washing gets rid of the initial grime and the second washing releases the underlying dirt. Then, once a day I use a product I've developed called Algae Deep Cleanse (see Sources) to gently remove dead skin cells from the skin's surface so that my skin can breathe. Since my skin is then thoroughly clean and the surface is clear of dead skin cells, there is no need for a toner. Some European skin care routines use heavy cleansers followed by strong, alcohol-based, perfumed toners to remove the grease left behind by the rich cleansers, but these toners dry the skin and cause enlarged pores. Many American skin care companies stress the use of soap and water, then toners to remove the soap scum. Regardless of the reasons for their use, toners made from alcohol dry out your skin, make your skin flake, and cause premature dehydration lines.

Moisturizing is essential right after you cleanse your skin. Even if you suffer from breakouts, your skin needs to be hydrated with a light and natural moisturizer. Light moisturizers don't contain mineral oil or paraffin wax and won't make your skin break out. After cleansing your face, I suggest using a few drops of Essential Oil Premoisturizer for your skin type (page 203) before applying a light moisturizer. It is also important to moisturize around your eyes, lids included. Use Vitamin E oil around your eyes and mouth just before going to bed.

If you experience breakouts, use a clay mask as a spot treatment over the blemishes to quickly help them heal. Clay is made up of silica, a trace mineral that helps refine the skin and encourages the body's own natural defense against bacteria.

Steaming

Steaming your pores once or twice a week over a bowl of hot water combined with a few sprigs or teaspoons of fresh or dried rosemary, thyme, lavender, or chamomile helps the skin heal more quickly from breakouts. Steaming encourages the pores to release impurities. For directions on steaming, see chapter 5.

MICRODERMABRASION BEWARE!

One of the least effective ways to improve your skin is with microdermabrasion. Many clients have told me about the disappointing results of this procedure. Microdermabrasion is a technique by which a facialist or dermatologist uses something similar to a tiny sandblaster to spray crystals all over the face. This is an abrasive way to remove dead skin cells. It is often done too aggressively and actually removes a layer of healthy skin. Microdermabrasion may cause microtears in the surface of the skin, leaving it much more vulnerable to the elements, especially the sun. It also changes the color of the skin to a waxy and somewhat abnormal tone. In addition, microdermabrasion does not remove blackheads or pimples.

Dry Skin Brushing

Dry skin brushing, in which you brush your whole body with a natural-bristle body brush or loofah, stimulates the circulation of blood and lymphatic fluid and helps eliminate dry, flaky skin and toxins. I have found it to be beneficial in minimizing cellulite. Dry-brush the entire body before bathing three times a week. Use a dry brush, a dry loofah sponge, or loofah gloves, which you can find in almost any bath and body store. Use short, brisk strokes, do not wet the brush, and always start at your feet and work your way up the body.

1. Start at your ankles and work your way up the legs, front and back.

2. Brush your abdomen clockwise, then your lower back toward your abdomen, and up your sternum toward your clavicle or collarbone.

3. Raise your arms above your head and stroke toward your armpit. Reach over your shoulder for the top of your back and brush in the direction of your collarbone again. Lightly brush your breasts in a clockwise direction.

4. Your skin should turn very pink, indicating increased circulation of the lymph and blood.

Toss loofah gloves right into the washing machine. For sanitizing other loofahs and brushes, wash them with 1 part bleach or "green" antibacterial detergent to 10 parts water in the sink and rinse thoroughly. Air-dry them.

Baths

There's no better place to alleviate fatigue, relax, reflect, and rejuvenate your body than in the bathtub. Sitting in the tub is also a perfect time to apply a balancing mask (page 197) to your face and neck.

You can help the detoxification process along by treating yourself once a week to detoxification baths using Epsom salts, organic apple cider vinegar, essential oils, or my Algae Fine Powder (see Sources). These are all gentle, natural detoxifiers that help the skin release its impurities. The following baths are not only therapeutic, they are powerful enough to help improve skin, too.

For all baths:

- Use very warm water but never too hot. Hot water causes your skin to lose elasticity, become dry, and is not good for your capillaries.

- Soak for 30 to 40 minutes a minimum of once a week.

- Sip a cup of herbal tea during each bath.

- Take a cool shower after each bath or rinse well to wash toxins from the surface of your skin.

- Be sure to disinfect and wash the tub before and after each use.

Apple Cider Vinegar Bath

This bath leaves you relishing in your positive energy and good vibrations! It lightens a bad mood and alleviates depression, negative energy, and emotional stress.

Add a minimum of 2 cups organic apple cider vinegar to running water.

Epsom Salt Bath

Epsom salts have been used for years as both a healing agent for minor sprains and strains and also to draw impurities out of the body through perspiration. This bath helps relieve muscle tension and fatigue.

Add 2 cups Epsom salts to running water. And for extra relaxation, also add ½ teaspoon of your favorite essential oil.

Essential Oil Bath

Certain essential oils can help to relieve tension in the body as well as soften your skin.

Combine 2 ounces macadamia nut oil with ¼ teaspoon of one of the following essential oils: lavender, rosemary, clary sage, or thyme. After mixing well, add to running water.

Algae Fine Powder Bath

I have found that my Algae Fine Powder (see Sources) reduces the effects of water retention and the appearance of cellulite (which contains 90 percent water).

Add 2 tablespoons Algae Fine Powder to running bath water.

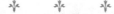

All of these practices, including a healthy diet, sufficient water intake, deep breathing, exercise, and skin treatments, will yield tremendous results in both the quality of your skin and your overall health. There is no end to the benefits you can achieve through detoxification. You'll feel better, look better, and have more energy. But remember, detoxification is only the beginning. A healthy lifestyle is an ongoing process that needs daily attention and care.

Aside from adopting a good skin care regimen and eating the right foods for your body, there are a number of habits you should begin incorporating into your routine to help the detoxification process take root in your life, your body, and your skin.

When you wake up: Floss and brush your teeth. Use a tongue cleaner to clean any bacteria from your tongue.

Detoxifying beverages: Drink one of the following beverages each morning before you eat. Feel free to alternate.

One large glass of spring water combined with the juice from one-half lemon, which supplies nutrients that assist in detoxification

One large glass of spring water combined with the juice from one-half lemon and 1 tablespoon olive oil, which acts as a gentle digestive lubricant

One large glass of spring water combined with 2 tablespoons organic apple cider vinegar and 2 tablespoons raw local honey

Now that you have been given the tools for better, more radiant skin, the next chapter will help you jump-start your detoxification process.

THREE

The 7-Day Plan
for Radiant Skin

In previous chapters, I explained how your diet directly impacts the health of your skin and how important exercise, breathing, skin care, and attitude are for a truly healthy body. In this chapter, you will learn how to put all of that information into practice. The following step-by-step, day-by-day cleansing program is designed to jump-start a healthier way of living and eating. It will improve your quality of life by detoxifying your system, increasing energy, and ultimately giving you a radiant, glowing complexion. Remember, this cleanse is meant to honor your body, so take pride in what you are giving it as opposed to what you think you are taking away. *The Ciminelli Solution* teaches you to pay attention to your body's real needs by finding the right balance of diet, exercise, and natural beauty care products. You are working to achieve good health the natural way and to improve your overall quality of life.

Caring for Your Skin Type

The 7-Day Plan for detoxification is designed to accommodate different skin types, so you need to determine yours. There are five basic skin types, and although no two people are alike, generally your skin is going to fall into one of these categories: normal, dry, oily, combination, or sensitive.

Normal skin has small to medium pores and good elasticity. In the 30 years that I've been in the field of skin care, I have never seen anyone with truly "normal" skin. Most people tend to have combination skin, with both oily and dry zones.

Dry skin is dull, tight, crinkly, brittle, and rough to the touch. It can flake and even itch. You may have fine lines and premature wrinkling. Skin is considered dry if it's dehydrated due to a lack of water intake or a lack of healthy oils, fat, and minerals in the diet. It can also be dry from overexposure to the sun. Dehydrated skin is the simplest to treat because all you need to do is increase your water intake, eat more green leafy vegetables, and adjust your diet to include foods that are rich in water such as fruits and vegetables like melons and cucumbers. Do this on a daily basis and within 1 week you'll see a difference. Even the fine lines, especially around the mouth and eye areas, will begin to diminish slightly. That's because the skin around the eye area is very tender and thin, and moisture escapes easily because of the lack of sebaceous glands, which produce natural oils. People who don't include enough healthy fats in their diet quickly show their age, especially around the eyes, mouth, and neck areas and eventually on the rest of the body.

Aside from diet, remember that dryness can be caused by soap, alcohol-based astringents, and skin care products that contain mineral oil and paraffin wax. People with dry skin should always use a natural moisturizer twice a day after cleansing. These products should contain pure essential oils, vitamins, and seaweed, if possible, which is rich in minerals, trace elements, and natural amino acids. Don't be tempted by glycolic acids. They tend to thin the skin and make it more susceptible to sun damage and premature aging. In addition to daily cleansing and moisturizing, dry skin will respond to a weekly at-home facial.

1. Steam your face with lavender- or chamomile-infused hot water for a few minutes (page 196).

2. Apply Avocado and Lemon Juice Mask (page 200) or spread 1 tablespoon raw organic honey in a thin layer on your face (avoiding the eyes and lips). Rinse the mask or honey off after 20 minutes with cool water. Gently dry your face with a clean towel.

3. Apply a thin layer of Essential Oil Premoisturizer for Dry Skin (page 203) on your face and neck. Finish by applying a natural moisturizer of your choice, allowing 5 minutes for it to absorb before applying makeup.

Oily skin tends to be shiny, greasy to the touch, and prone to blemishes and blackheads. Pores are larger and the skin feels thick rather than firm, similar to the texture and look of an orange. Oily skin is caused by a poor diet and hormonal imbalance, which is why you so often see teens with acne. It can also be the result of a diet rich in animal fats and protein, sugar, coffee, soda, and other junk foods. If you use greasy, heavy moisturizers that contain paraffin or mineral oil, you could misdiagnose your skin as oily. People with oily skin should cleanse the face three times a day in the beginning to help prevent clogged pores and reduce blemishes. Even though the skin is oily, it should be moisturized after it is cleansed with Essential Oil Premoisturizer (page 203) made with lemon, lemongrass, and tea tree oils. These oils have antibacterial properties and help purify the natural oil present in the skin's oil glands and pores. Oily skin also benefits from a weekly at-home facial.

1. Thoroughly wash your face with a gel cleanser.

2. Steam your face with rosemary-infused hot water for a few minutes to cleanse your pores.

3. With clean hands, wrap a tissue around your fingers and gently apply pressure to each side of any pimple or clogged pore to extract the waste. If you are unable to remove the waste on your first attempt, resteam your face for a few more minutes and try again, until the waste has been removed. Wipe your face with peroxide or witch hazel applied to a cotton ball to remove any residue.

4. Apply 1 teaspoon of a clay mask combined with ¼ teaspoon Oily Skin Essential Oil Premoisturizer (page 203), and leave

it on your face (avoiding eyes and lips) for about 15 minutes to tighten and restore the skin. Rinse off the mask with cool water and pat the skin dry with a clean towel.

5. Apply a thin layer of Oily Skin Essential Oil Premoisturizer (page 203) on your face, and Essential Oil Premoisturizer for dry skin on your neck.

6. Finish by applying a paraffin-free and mineral oil–free natural lightweight moisturizer of your choice. Allow 5 minutes for it to absorb before applying makeup.

7. During the week, spot treat any blemishes with a dab of a clay mask before bed. Repeat this facial once a week for several weeks to clear oily skin.

❧ PRACTICAL TIPS FOR GOOD SKIN CARE AT HOME ❧

- Wash your hands well with a gel cleanser—not soap—and warm water before washing your face.
- Wash your face with warm water and rinse with cool, then repeat.
- Use a clean towel every time you wash your face.
- Use natural skin care products that do not contain mineral oil, paraffin wax, perfume, or specially denatured (SD) alcohol.
- Steam your pores once a week and follow with a mask.
- Moisturize around your eyes and lips with vitamin E oil at night to keep these delicate areas moist and young-looking.
- Apply your moisturizer over damp skin.
- If you do break out, make sure that you get right back on track with good eating habits, proper breathing, and drinking enough water, which will all help with the elimination of toxins.

Combination skin is probably the most common skin type. With combination skin, oily skin will show up in the T-zone, the area consisting of the forehead, nose, and chin, while the cheeks and eye area will remain dry or normal. This type of skin is the easiest to deal with because as soon as you bring it into balance with the right cleanser and moisturizers, it will become radiant and beautiful. Remember to wash your face with warm water and a gentle gel cleanser twice a day. Rinse with cool water, pat dry, and immediately premoisturize by applying Dry Skin Essential Oil Premoisturizer (page 203) to the periphery of your face and Oily Skin Essential Oil Premoisturizer (see page 203) to your T-zone area. Follow with a light moisturizer. This basic cleansing and moisturizing treatment will help balance the dry and oily parts of the face.

Combination skin benefits from a weekly at-home facial. Since combination skin contains both dry and oily components, apply the weekly at-home facial for dry skin to the periphery of your face and the at-home facial for oily skin to your T-zone area for complete and balanced coverage.

With *sensitive skin,* you often see an increased number of broken capillaries toward the surface. It is also highly susceptible to the environment and to chemicals in cleansers, moisturizers, sunscreen, and makeup. People with sensitive skin cannot rely on the "hypoallergenic" label on packaging because these products may contain unnatural and unhealthy ingredients such as perfume, alcohol, mineral oil, and paraffin wax. Stick with products that are healthy, natural, and nourishing. Look for skin care items that contain essential oils, vitamins, antioxidants and natural ingredients such as seaweed and algae. People with sensitive skin should also incorporate more good fats (page 13) into their diet and should try to avoid caffeine and spicy foods, which can irritate the system.

Wash your face in the morning and the evening with a natural cleansing milk rather than a gel-based cleanser. Cleansing milk is the most mild cleanser and will not irritate sensitive skin. Follow with a thin layer of Sensitive Skin Essential Oil Premoisturizer (page 203) and finish with a natural lightweight moisturizer. Sensitive skin can also benefit from a weekly at-home facial.

1. Steam your face with chamomile-infused hot water for a few minutes.

2. Apply a Honey–Bee Pollen Mask (page 197) or spread 1 tablespoon raw organic honey in a thin layer on your face. Rinse the mask or honey off after 20 minutes with cool water. Dry your face with a clean towel.

3. Apply a thin layer of Essential Oil Premoisturizer for Sensitive Skin (page 203) on your face and neck.

4. Finish by applying a natural moisturizer of your choice over damp skin.

Following the steps for your specific skin type in combination with a detoxifying diet and lifestyle will produce beautiful skin that will no longer require liquid foundation makeup. Instead, a quick dusting of translucent powder is all you will need to even out your skin tone. After a week of detoxifying skin care and diet, your skin will show vast improvement.

Now that you know which skin type you have and how to take care of it, you are about to embark on the 7-Day Plan. The 7-Day

Plan for Radiant Skin will help elevate your spirits, clear your mind, strengthen your body, reduce the size of your pores, and give you a more radiant, glowing complexion. Just remember, as with any food or exercise program, review this one with your health care professional.

❈ DAILY SKIN CARE PRACTICES FOR ❈ THE 7-DAY PLAN FOR DETOXIFICATION

In order to achieve maximum results from this detoxification plan, try to do these things on a daily basis:

- Brush and floss your teeth and scrape your tongue first thing in the morning.
- Wash your hands before you wash your face.
- Wash your face with a mild gel or milk cleanser and warm water twice a day.
- Never use soap, hot water, or extremely cold water on your face.
- Always pat your face dry. Do not rub.
- After cleansing your face, moisturize with an essential oil premoisturizer (page 203) and follow with a natural moisturizer that contains essential oils, vitamins, and nutrients derived from plants, algae, seaweed, and herbs. (Avoid moisturizers that contain paraffin, alcohol, or mineral oils.)

7-Day Plan for Radiant Skin

We start with the 7-Day Plan for Normal and Dry Skin Types. If you have oily or troubled skin (broken out), use the Alternate 7-Day Plan on page 80.

Whenever possible, try to eat organic fruits, vegetables, and protein. If you are unable to buy organic produce, be sure to wash your fruits and vegetables thoroughly (page 36) to remove surface pesticides or chemicals.

Remember that the way in which you eat is as important as what you eat. Never eat when you are agitated. Be sure to take some deep breaths to relax before eating. Eating in an agitated state can prevent proper digestion. Chew your food well. Drink 8 to 10 glasses of pure spring water every day.

Exercise and yoga also play a large role in the plan. If you are not used to doing exercise or yoga on a regular basis, start out doing a few minutes of each on Day 1, and increase the amount of time each day.

As you follow the 7-Day Plan, snack if you need to, but avoid junk food such as chips, candy, and soda. It's important to choose snacks that nourish, satisfy, and cleanse your system. The following do just that. Keep in mind that these snacks are optional. Try not to eat more than two servings of snacks per day. Eat less than the indicated quantity if desired but never more.

Healthy Snacks

1 cup blueberries, raspberries, strawberries, cherries, or grapes

1 cup fresh pomegranate seeds

2 carrots

2 celery ribs

1 cup peeled, seeded, and sliced cucumber

½ fennel bulb

¼ cup almonds (avoid for oily or troubled skin)

¼ cup macadamia nuts (avoid for oily or troubled skin)

¼ cup walnuts (avoid for oily or troubled skin)

¼ cup pecans (avoid for oily or troubled skin)

¼ cup raw or toasted pumpkin seeds

2–3 radishes

1 cup mixed raw vegetables with Yogurt Herb Dip (page 182)

½ small avocado (if your skin is dry)

Day 1

Upon Rising

Abdominal Massage (page 41)

Teeth and Tongue Brushing (page 41)

Dry Skin Brushing (page 46)

Cleanse and Moisturize Face (see page 52 for specific skin types)

Throughout the Day

Speed Walk or other Aerobic Activity (page 40) for 35–45 minutes

20-minute Yoga Routine (page 216)

Breakfast

8 ounces spring water combined with juice from ½ lemon (drink 15 minutes before eating breakfast)

1 cup organic goat's milk yogurt

1 cup mixed fresh berries *or* ½ cup mixed berries combined with ½ cup pomegranate seeds

1 teaspoon crushed bee pollen (page 99)

1 tablespoon ground flaxseeds (page 102)

1 cup herbal tea

Snack

1 serving of a Healthy Snack (page 60)

Lunch

8 ounces spring water combined with juice from ½ lemon
(drink 15 minutes before eating lunch)

1–2 cups Creamy Broccoli Soup (page 117)

2 cups Antioxidant Salad (page 122) *or* Cleansing Salad
(page 123)

1 tablespoon Lemon–Lime Olive Oil Dressing (page 177) *or*
Sherry Vinaigrette (page 178)

3 ounces chicken *or* turkey (see recipes on pages 130–140)

1 cup herbal tea

Snack

1 serving of a Healthy Snack (page 60)

Dinner

8 ounces spring water combined with juice from ½ lemon
(drink 15 minutes before eating dinner)

2 cups Antioxidant Salad (page 122) *or* Cleansing Salad (page 123)

1 tablespoon Lemon–Lime Olive Oil Dressing (page 177) *or* Sherry Vinaigrette (page 178)

4 ounces chicken *or* fish (see recipes on pages 130–151)

1 cup cooked vegetables of your choice (see pages 168–175)

1 cup herbal tea

Before Retiring

Cleanse and Moisturize Face (see page 52 for specific skin types)

1 cup Smooth Move and Chamomile Tea (page 230)

Deep Breathing (page 212)

Day 2

Upon Rising

Abdominal Massage (page 41)

Dry Skin Brushing (page 46)

Teeth and Tongue Brushing (page 41)

Steaming (see page 196 for steam baths for specific skin types)

Clay Mask Combined with Essential Oil Application (page 203)

Cleanse and Moisturize Face (see page 52 for specific skin types)

Throughout the Day

Speed Walk or other Aerobic Activity (page 40) for 35–45 minutes

20-minute Yoga Routine (page 216)

Breakfast

8 ounces spring water combined with juice from ½ lemon (drink 15 minutes before eating breakfast)

1–2 large organic eggs, scrambled in 1 teaspoon olive oil, topped with 1 tablespoon ground flaxseeds (page 102)

1 slice Ezekiel *or* sprouted grain bread, toasted and spread with ½ teaspoon olive oil

½ grapefruit

1 cup herbal tea

Snack

1 serving of a Healthy Snack (page 60)

Lunch

8 ounces spring water combined with juice from ½ lemon (drink 15 minutes before eating lunch)

2 cups Antioxidant Salad (page 122) *or* Cleansing Salad (page 123)

1 tablespoon Lemon-Lime Olive Oil Dressing (page 177) *or*
Sherry Vinaigrette (page 178)

3 ounces chicken *or* turkey (see recipes on pages 130–140)

½ avocado drizzled with fresh lemon juice and a pinch of sea salt

1 cup herbal tea

Snack

1 serving of a Healthy Snack (page 60)

Dinner

8 ounces spring water combined with juice from ½ lemon
(drink 15 minutes before eating dinner)

1–2 cups Tuscan Bean Soup (page 114)

2 cups Antioxidant Salad (page 122) *or* Cleansing Salad (page 123)

1 tablespoon Lemon-Lime Olive Oil Dressing (page 177) *or*
Sherry Vinaigrette (page 178)

4 ounces fish *or* chicken (see recipes on pages 130–151)

1 cup cooked vegetables of your choice (pages 168–175)

1 cup herbal tea

Before Retiring

Epsom Salt Bath (page 48), Apple Cider Vinegar Bath (page 48),
or Algae Fine Powder Bath (page 49)

Cleanse and Moisturize Face (see page 52 for specific skin types)

1 cup Smooth Move and Chamomile Tea (page 230)

Deep Breathing (page 212)

Day 3

Upon Rising

Abdominal Massage (page 41)

Teeth and Tongue Brushing (page 41)

Dry Skin Brushing (page 46)

Cleanse and Moisturize Face (see page 52 for specific skin types)

Throughout the Day

Speed Walk or other Aerobic Activity (page 40) for 35–45 minutes

20-minute Yoga Routine (page 216)

Breakfast

8 ounces spring water combined with juice from ½ lemon (drink 15 minutes before eating breakfast)

1 cup organic goat's milk yogurt

1 cup mixed fresh berries or ½ cup mixed berries combined with ½ cup pomegranate seeds

1 teaspoon crushed bee pollen (page 99)

1 tablespoon ground flaxseeds (page 102)

1 cup herbal tea

Snack

1 serving of a Healthy Snack (page 60)

Lunch

8 ounces spring water combined with juice from ½ lemon (drink 15 minutes before eating lunch)

1–2 cups Tuscan Bean Soup (page 114)

2 cups Antioxidant Salad (page 122) *or* Cleansing Salad (page 123)

1 tablespoon Lemon–Lime Olive Oil Dressing (page 177) *or* Sherry Vinaigrette (page 178)

3 ounces fish *or* chicken (see recipes on pages 130–151)

1 cup herbal tea

Snack

1 serving of a Healthy Snack (page 60)

Dinner

8 ounces spring water combined with juice from ½ lemon (drink 15 minutes before eating dinner)

2 cups Antioxidant Salad (page 122) *or* Cleansing Salad (page 123)

1 tablespoon Lemon–Lime Olive Oil Dressing (page 177) *or* Sherry Vinaigrette (page 178)

4 ounces fish (see recipes on pages 142–151)

1 cup cooked vegetables of your choice (see pages 168–175)

1 cup herbal tea

Before Retiring

Epsom Salt Bath (page 48), Apple Cider Vinegar Bath (page 48), or Algae Fine Powder Bath (page 49)

Clay Mask Combined with Essential Oil Application (page 203)

❧ DAY 3: PROGRESS CHECK ❧

By now, your stomach should feel smaller and you should be feeling lighter and cleaner from the inside out. Remember that the 7-Day Plan is just a jump-start to get you on the right track. Be sure to include both cooked and raw vegetables, and make sure that you vary your choices with vegetables grown above the ground and below the ground for optimal health. Your food choices should be colorful whenever possible. Eat slowly and chew each mouthful very carefully to stimulate and aid digestion and elimination.

Cleanse and Moisturize Face (see page 52 for specific skin types)

1 cup Smooth Move and Chamomile Tea (page 230)

Deep Breathing (page 212)

Day 4

Upon Rising

Abdominal Massage (page 41)

Teeth and Tongue Brushing (page 41)

Dry Skin Brushing (page 46)

Cleanse and Moisturize Face (see page 52 for specific skin types)

Throughout the Day

Speed Walk or other Aerobic Activity (page 40) for 35–45 minutes

20-minute Yoga Routine (page 216)

Breakfast

8 ounces spring water combined with juice from ½ lemon (drink 15 minutes before eating breakfast)

1–2 large organic eggs, scrambled in 1 teaspoon olive oil, topped with 1 tablespoon ground flaxseeds (page 102)

1 slice Ezekiel *or* sprouted grain bread, toasted and spread with ½ teaspoon olive oil

½ avocado drizzled with fresh lemon juice and a pinch of sea salt

1 cup herbal tea

Snack

1 serving of a Healthy Snack (page 60)

Lunch

8 ounces spring water combined with juice from ½ lemon (drink 15 minutes before eating lunch)

1–2 cups Creamy Broccoli Soup (page 117)

2 cups Antioxidant Salad (page 122) *or* Cleansing Salad (page 123)

1 tablespoon Lemon-Lime Olive Oil Dressing (page 177) *or* Sherry Vinaigrette (page 178)

3 ounces chicken (see recipes on pages 130–136)

1 cup herbal tea

Snack

1 serving of a Healthy Snack (page 60)

Dinner

8 ounces spring water combined with juice from ½ lemon (drink 15 minutes before eating dinner)

2 cups Antioxidant Salad (page 122) *or* Cleansing Salad (page 123)

1 tablespoon Lemon–Lime Olive Oil Dressing (page 177) *or* Sherry Vinaigrette (page 178)

4 ounces fish (see recipes on pages 142–151)

1 cup cooked vegetables of your choice (pages 168–175)

1 cup herbal tea

Before Retiring

Epsom Salt Bath (page 48), Apple Cider Vinegar Bath (page 48), or Algae Fine Powder Bath (page 49)

Clay Mask Combined with Essential Oil Application (page 203)

Cleanse and Moisturize Face (see page 52 for specific skin types)

1 cup Smooth Move and Chamomile Tea (page 71)

Deep Breathing (page 212)

Day 5

Upon Rising

Abdominal Massage (page 41)

Teeth and Tongue Brushing (page 41)

Dry Skin Brushing (page 46)

Cleanse and Moisturize Face (see page 52 for specific skin types)

Throughout the Day

Speed Walk or other Aerobic Activity (page 40) for 35–45 minutes

20-minute Yoga Routine (page 216)

Breakfast

8 ounces spring water combined with juice from ½ lemon (drink 15 minutes before eating breakfast)

1 cup organic goat's milk yogurt

1 cup mixed fresh berries *or* ½ cup mixed berries combined with ½ cup pomegranate seeds

1 teaspoon crushed bee pollen (page 99)

1 tablespoon ground flaxseeds (page 102)

1 cup herbal tea

Snack

1 serving of a Healthy Snack (page 60)

Lunch

8 ounces spring water combined with juice from ½ lemon
(drink 15 minutes before eating lunch)

1–2 cups Tuscan Bean Soup (see page 114)

2 cups Antioxidant Salad (page 122) *or* Cleansing Salad
(page 123)

1 tablespoon Lemon–Lime Olive Oil Dressing (page 177) *or*
Sherry Vinaigrette (page 178)

3 ounces fish *or* chicken (see recipes on pages 130–151)

1 cup herbal tea

Snack

1 serving of a Healthy Snack (page 60)

Dinner

8 ounces spring water combined with juice from ½ lemon
(drink 15 minutes before eating dinner)

2 cups Antioxidant Salad (page 122) *or* Cleansing Salad
(page 123)

1 tablespoon Lemon–Lime Olive Oil Dressing (page 177) *or* Sherry Vinaigrette (page 178)

4 ounces fish (see recipes on pages 142–151)

1 cup cooked vegetables of your choice (pages 168–175)

1 cup herbal tea

Before Retiring

Epsom Salt Bath (see page 48), Apple Cider Vinegar Bath (see page 48), or Algae Fine Powder Bath (see page 49)

Cleanse and Moisturize Face (see page 52 for specific skin types)

1 cup Smooth Move and Chamomile Tea (see page 230)

Deep Breathing (see page 212)

❖ DAY 5: PROGRESS CHECK ❖

If you are eating slowly enough and drinking your water, the amount of food should satisfy you. Remember that your stomach is as big as your closed fist. The golden rule of healthy eating is one-third air, one-third liquid, and one-third thoroughly chewed food in your stomach. The air provides the room for the food to be tossed around in the stomach while it is being coated with digestive enzymes. This process can only happen when you are in the calm stage of rest. Never take it for granted that the food you are eating is going to automatically be digested. We have to earn our health and beauty. Breathing slowly and deeply keeps you calm, relaxed, and centered.

Day 6

Upon Rising

Abdominal Massage (page 41)

Teeth and Tongue Brushing (page 41)

Dry Skin Brushing (page 46)

Cleanse and Moisturize Face (see page 52 for specific skin types)

Throughout the Day

Speed Walk or other Aerobic Activity (page 40) for
35–45 minutes

20-minute Yoga Routine (page 216)

Breakfast

8 ounces spring water combined with juice from ½ lemon
(drink 15 minutes before eating breakfast)

1–2 large organic eggs, scrambled in 1 teaspoon olive oil, topped
with 1 tablespoon ground flaxseeds (page 102)

1 slice Ezekiel *or* sprouted grain bread, toasted and spread with
½ teaspoon olive oil

½ avocado drizzled with fresh lemon juice and a pinch of sea salt

1 cup herbal tea

Snack

1 serving of a Healthy Snack (page 60)

Lunch

8 ounces spring water combined with juice from ½ lemon (drink 15 minutes before eating lunch)

2 cups Antioxidant Salad (page 122) *or* Cleansing Salad (page 123)

1 tablespoon Lemon–Lime Olive Oil Dressing (page 177) *or* Sherry Vinaigrette (page 178)

3 ounces chicken (see recipes on pages 130–136)

1 cup herbal tea

Snack

1 serving of a Healthy Snack (page 60)

Dinner

8 ounces spring water combined with juice from ½ lemon (drink 15 minutes before eating dinner)

1–2 cups Creamy Broccoli Soup (page 117)

4 ounces fish (see recipes on pages 142–151)

1 cup cooked vegetables of your choice (pages 168–175)

1 cup herbal tea

Cleanse and Moisturize Face (see page 52 for specific skin types)

1 cup Smooth Move and Chamomile Tea (page 230)

Deep Breathing (page 212)

Day 7

Upon Rising

Abdominal Massage (page 41)

Teeth and Tongue Brushing (page 41)

Dry Skin Brushing Massage (page 46)

Cleanse and Moisturize Face (see page 52 for specific skin types)

Throughout the Day

Speed Walk or other Aerobic Activity (page 40) for 35–45 minutes

20-minute Yoga Routine (page 216)

Breakfast

8 ounces spring water combined with juice from ½ lemon (drink 15 minutes before eating breakfast)

1 cup organic goat's milk yogurt

1 cup mixed fresh berries *or* ½ cup mixed berries combined with ½ cup pomegranate seeds

1 teaspoon crushed bee pollen (page 99)

1 tablespoon ground flaxseeds (page 102)

1 cup herbal tea

Snack

1 serving of a Healthy Snack (page 60)

Lunch

8 ounces spring water combined with juice from ½ lemon (drink 15 minutes before eating lunch)

2 cups Antioxidant Salad (page 122) *or* Cleansing Salad (page 123)

1 tablespoon Lemon-Lime Olive Oil Dressing (page 177) *or* Sherry Vinaigrette (page 178)

3 ounces chicken *or* fish (see recipes on pages 130–151)

1 cup herbal tea

Snack

1 serving of a Healthy Snack (page 60)

Dinner

8 ounces spring water combined with juice from ½ lemon (drink 15 minutes before eating dinner)

1–2 cups Tuscan Bean Soup (page 114)

2 cups Antioxidant Salad (page 122) *or* Cleansing Salad (page 123)

1 tablespoon Lemon–Lime Olive Oil Dressing (page 177) *or* Sherry Vinaigrette (page 178)

4 ounces fish *or* chicken (see recipes on pages 130–151)

1 cup herbal tea

Before Retiring

Epsom Salt Bath (page 48), Apple Cider Vinegar Bath (page 48), or Algae Fine Powder Bath (page 49)

Cleanse and Moisturize Face (see page 52 for specific skin types)

1 cup Smooth Move and Chamomile Tea (page 230)

Deep Breathing (page 212)

Those with oily or troubled (broken out) skin should follow this alternate food plan that is lower in fats and higher in protein. The addition of freshly extracted homemade juices (page 186) help benefit the immune system and aid in cleansing the body. Acidophilus Probiotic (see Sources) is a healthy colonic bacteria that helps your body reduce the levels of harmful bacteria and yeasts in the intestines. When the levels of harmful bacteria are out of balance, gas, bloating, toxicity, and constipation may result. Acidophilus Probiotic helps restore a proper intestinal balance, better elimination, and therefore better skin quality.

Remember to follow the same exercise and skin care routines listed in the 7-Day Plan for Normal and Dry Skin Types.

Day 1

Breakfast

8 ounces spring water combined with juice from ½ lemon (drink 15 minutes before eating breakfast)

1 tablespoon (any flavor) liquid Acidophilus Probiotic (see Sources)

8 ounces freshly extracted juice of your choice (page 186)

1½ cups high-fiber bran cereal with 1 tablespoon ground flaxseeds (page 102)

¾ cup unsweetened soy milk

½ cup blueberries *or* ½ cup pomegranate seeds

1 large poached organic egg

1 cup herbal tea

Snack

8 ounces freshly extracted juice of your choice (page 186)

Lunch

8 ounces spring water combined with juice from ½ lemon (drink 15 minutes before eating lunch)

2 cups Antioxidant Salad (page 122) *or* Cleansing Salad (page 123)

1 tablespoon Lemon-Lime Olive Oil Dressing (page 177) *or* Sherry Vinaigrette (page 178)

4 ounces chicken (see recipes on pages 130–136)

1 cup herbal tea

Snack

1 serving of a Healthy Snack (page 60)

Dinner

8 ounces spring water combined with juice from ½ lemon
(drink 15 minutes before eating dinner)

2 cups Antioxidant Salad (page 122) *or* Cleansing Salad
(page 123)

1 tablespoon Lemon–Lime Olive Oil Dressing (page 177) *or*
Sherry Vinaigrette (page 178)

4 ounces chicken *or* fish (see recipes on pages 130–151)

1 cup cooked vegetables of your choice (pages 168–175)

1 cup herbal tea

Day 2

Breakfast

8 ounces spring water combined with juice from ½ lemon
(drink 15 minutes before eating breakfast)

1 tablespoon (any flavor) liquid Acidophilus Probiotic (see
Sources)

8 ounces freshly extracted juice of your choice (page 186)

1–2 large organic eggs, scrambled in 1 teaspoon olive oil, topped
with 1 tablespoon ground flaxseeds (page 102), *or* 2 cups Tofu
Casserole (page 153)

1 slice Ezekiel *or* sprouted grain bread, toasted and spread with ½ teaspoon olive oil

1 cup herbal tea

Snack

8 ounces freshly extracted juice of your choice (page 186)

Lunch

8 ounces spring water combined with juice from ½ lemon (drink 15 minutes before eating lunch)

2 cups Antioxidant Salad (page 122) *or* Cleansing Salad (page 123)

1 tablespoon Lemon–Lime Olive Oil Dressing (page 177) *or* Sherry Vinaigrette (page 178)

4 ounces fish (see recipes on pages 142–151)

1 cup herbal tea

Snack

1 serving of a Healthy Snack (page 60)

Dinner

8 ounces spring water combined with juice from ½ lemon (drink 15 minutes before eating dinner)

1–2 cups Mung Bean Vegetable Soup (page 116)

2 cups Antioxidant Salad (page 122) *or* Cleansing Salad (page 123)

1 tablespoon Lemon–Lime Olive Oil Dressing (page 177) *or* Sherry Vinaigrette (page 178)

4 ounces fish *or* chicken

1 cup herbal tea

Day 3

Breakfast

8 ounces spring water combined with juice from ½ lemon (drink 15 minutes before eating breakfast)

1 tablespoon (any flavor) liquid Acidophilus Probiotic (see Sources)

8 ounces freshly extracted juice of your choice (page 186)

1½ cups high-fiber cereal with 1 tablespoon ground flaxseed (page 102)

¾ cup unsweetened soy milk

1 large poached organic egg

1 cup herbal tea

Snack

8 ounces freshly extracted juice of your choice (page 186)

Lunch

8 ounces spring water combined with juice from ½ lemon (drink 15 minutes before eating lunch)

2 cups Antioxidant Salad (page 122) *or* Cleansing Salad (page 123)

1 tablespoon Lemon–Lime Olive Oil Dressing (page 177) *or* Sherry Vinaigrette (page 178)

4 ounces fish *or* chicken (see recipes on pages 130–151)

1 cup herbal tea

Snack

1 serving of a Healthy Snack (page 60)

Dinner

8 ounces spring water combined with juice from ½ lemon (drink 15 minutes before eating dinner)

1–2 cups Adzuki Bean Soup (page 112)

2 cups Antioxidant Salad (page 122) *or* Cleansing Salad (page 123)

1 tablespoon Lemon-Lime Olive Oil Dressing (page 177) *or* Sherry Vinaigrette (page 178)

4 ounces fish *or* chicken *or* turkey (see recipes on pages 130–151)

1 cup herbal tea

Day 4

Breakfast

8 ounces spring water combined with juice from ½ lemon (drink 15 minutes before eating breakfast)

1 tablespoon (any flavor) liquid Acidophilus Probiotic (see Sources)

8 ounces freshly extracted juice of your choice (page 186)

1–2 large organic eggs, scrambled in 1 teaspoon olive oil, topped with 1 tablespoon ground flaxseeds (page 102), *or* 1 cup Tofu Casserole (page 153)

1 slice Exekiel *or* sprouted grain bread, toasted and spread with ½ teaspoon olive oil

1 cup herbal tea

Snack

8 ounces freshly extracted juice of your choice (page 186)

Lunch

8 ounces spring water combined with juice from ½ lemon (drink 15 minutes before eating lunch)

2 cups Antioxidant Salad (page 122) *or* Cleansing Salad (page 123)

1 tablespoon Lemon–Lime Olive Oil Dressing (page 177) *or* Sherry Vinaigrette (page 178)

4 ounces fish *or* chicken *or* turkey (see recipes on pages 130–151)

1 cup herbal tea

Snack

1 serving of a Healthy Snack (page 60)

Dinner

8 ounces spring water combined with juice from ½ lemon (drink 15 minutes before eating dinner)

1–2 cups Mung Bean Vegetable Soup (page 116)

2 cups Antioxidant Salad (page 122) *or* Cleansing Salad (page 123)

1 tablespoon Lemon–Lime Olive Oil Dressing (page 177) *or* Sherry Vinaigrette (page 178)

4 ounces fish *or* chicken *or* turkey (see recipes on pages 130–151)

1 cup herbal tea

Day 5

Breakfast

8 ounces spring water combined with juice from ½ lemon (drink 15 minutes before eating breakfast)

1 tablespoon (any flavor) liquid Acidophilus Probiotic (see Sources)

8 ounces freshly extracted juice of your choice (page 186)

1½ cups high-fiber cereal with 1 tablespoon ground flaxseeds (page 102)

¾ cup unsweetened soy milk

1 large poached organic egg

1 cup herbal tea

Snack

8 ounces freshly extracted juice of your choice (page 186)

Lunch

8 ounces spring water combined with juice from ½ lemon (drink 15 minutes before eating lunch)

2 cups Antioxidant Salad (page 122) *or* Cleansing Salad (page 123)

1 tablespoon Lemon-Lime Olive Oil Dressing (page 177) *or* Sherry Vinaigrette (page 178)

4 ounces fish *or* chicken *or* turkey (see recipes on pages 130–151)

1 cup herbal tea

Snack

1 serving of a Healthy Snack (page 60)

Dinner

8 ounces spring water combined with juice from ½ lemon (drink 15 minutes before eating dinner)

1–2 cups Adzuki Bean Soup (page 112)

2 cups Antioxidant Salad (page 122) *or* Cleansing Salad (page 123)

1 tablespoon Lemon-Lime Olive Oil Dressing (page 177) *or* Sherry Vinaigrette (page 178)

4 ounces fish *or* chicken *or* turkey (see recipes on pages 130–151)

1 cup herbal tea

Day 6

Breakfast

8 ounces spring water combined with juice from ½ lemon (drink 15 minutes before eating breakfast)

1 tablespoon (any flavor) liquid Acidophilus Probiotic (see Sources)

8 ounces freshly extracted juice of your choice (page 186)

1–2 large organic eggs, scrambled in 1 teaspoon of olive oil, topped with 1 tablespoon ground flaxseeds (page 102), *or* 1 cup Tofu Casserole (page 153)

1 cup herbal tea

Snack

8 ounces freshly extracted juice of your choice (see page 186)

Lunch

8 ounces spring water combined with juice from ½ lemon (drink 15 minutes before eating lunch)

2 cups Antioxidant Salad (page 122) *or* Cleansing Salad (page 123)

1 tablespoon Lemon–Lime Olive Oil Dressing (page 177) *or* Sherry Vinaigrette (page 178)

4 ounces fish *or* chicken *or* turkey (see recipes on pages 130–151)

1 cup herbal tea

Snack

1 serving of a Healthy Snack (page 60)

Dinner

8 ounces spring water combined with juice from ½ lemon (drink 15 minutes before eating dinner)

1–2 cups Mung Bean Vegetable Soup (page 116)

2 cups Antioxidant Salad (page 122) *or* Cleansing Salad (page 123)

1 tablespoon Lemon-Lime Olive Oil Dressing (page 177) *or* Sherry Vinaigrette (page 178)

4 ounces fish *or* chicken *or* turkey (see recipes on pages 130–151)

1 cup herbal tea

Day 7

Breakfast

8 ounces spring water combined with juice from ½ lemon (drink 15 minutes before eating breakfast)

1 tablespoon (any flavor) liquid Acidophilus Probiotic (see Sources)

8 ounces freshly extracted juice of your choice (see page 186)

1–2 large organic eggs, scrambled in 1 teaspoon of olive oil, topped with 1 tablespoon ground flaxseeds (page 102), *or*

1 cup Tofu Casserole (page 153)

1 slice Ezekiel *or* sprouted grain bread, toasted and spread with ½ teaspoon olive oil

1 cup herbal tea

Snack

8 ounces freshly extracted vegetable juice of your choice (see page 186)

Lunch

8 ounces spring water combined with juice from ½ lemon (drink 15 minutes before eating lunch)

2 cups Antioxidant Salad (page 122) *or* Cleansing Salad (page 123)

1 tablespoon Lemon-Lime Olive Oil Dressing (page 177) *or*
Sherry Vinaigrette (page 178)

4 ounces fish *or* chicken *or* turkey (see recipes on pages 130–151)

1 cup herbal tea

Snack

1 serving of a Healthy Snack (page 60)

Dinner

8 ounces spring water combined with juice from ½ lemon
(drink 15 minutes before eating dinner)

1–2 cups Adzuki Bean Soup (page 112)

2 cups Antioxidant Salad (page 122) *or* Cleansing Salad
(page 123)

1 tablespoon Lemon-Lime Olive Oil Dressing (page 177) *or*
Sherry Vinaigrette (page 178)

4 ounces fish *or* chicken *or* turkey (see recipes on pages 130–151)

1 cup herbal tea

❈   ❈   ❈

Congratulations. You have just treated your body to a wonderful internal cleansing and nourishing process. This will result in healthier skin, a smaller stomach, and the beginning of a new internal and external health. You should also know that this type of eating helps curb the craving for processed sugar and useless carbs that pack on the pounds. Even though you are eating fruits that contain sugar, they are natural sugars and balanced with essential enzymes, vitamins, and fiber.

You can stay on this eating plan as long as you like—just incorporate 2 more ounces of protein with lunch or dinner. If desired, you can also add 1 cup of cooked basmati rice, short-grain brown rice, millet, or quinoa at lunch each day. If you do choose to incorporate these healthy starches, try and exercise a bit more to burn the extra calories.

FOUR

Eating Right for a Lifetime of Beauty

Now that you have completed the 7-Day Plan and are well on your way to a healthy, balanced, and detoxified body, there are some things you need to do to maintain this level of health and beauty. While the 7-Day Plan jump-started your body, in order to keep your skin clear and radiant, you must continue to eat beneficial foods filled with vitamins, minerals, and nutrients, and avoid toxic elements including animal fats, processed food, cow's milk dairy products, white sugar, white flour, soda, and coffee.

I encourage you to prepare as many of your meals at home as you can so that you know exactly what is going into each dish. Restaurants often add huge amounts of salt, sugar, and fat to enhance flavor, which adds calories as well. Cooking and eating at home can be a labor of love for both yourself and those you cook for.

Whether you are a novice or a seasoned cook, the recipes in this chapter will appeal for both their ease of preparation and taste. These recipes for soups, salads, proteins, legumes, vegetables, juices, and smoothies will get you started. Remember that no matter what recipe you are preparing, always try and cook with organic, local, seasonal ingredients.

In addition to a selection of healthful and delicious recipes, this chapter provides information on how to set up your kitchen to make it a welcoming place to cook, how to set up and keep a healthy pantry, how to shop healthy, and how to read food labels properly to ensure that you are buying the best-quality foods.

The Working Kitchen

The kitchen is undoubtedly the heart of any home. It is where we all tend to gather not just to eat meals but also to chat, hang out, and be together. However, for an inexperienced or insecure cook, the kitchen can be a source of tension. But if you have the right ingredients and a few key pieces of kitchen equipment on hand, you can prepare meals in very little time. The trick is to keep your kitchen organized and your pantry stocked. This will help you approach food and food preparation with ease, joy, purity, and a new appreciation for flavor. Even with my busy schedule, cooking has become less of a chore and more something I look forward to—an expression of love.

The best way to detoxify your kitchen and allow for a well-stocked, healthy pantry is to first take an inventory of its contents. Getting rid of toxic processed foods, out-of-date spices (those more than a year old) and condiments, rancid nuts and seeds, broken kitchen utensils, and scratched nonstick pans is a must. Also be sure to get in the habit of laundering hand towels, dish towels, oven mitts, potholders, and aprons on a regular basis to avoid harmful bacteria.

At this point, you may also want to take stock of your cookware. There are a few basic items that will help you cook with ease. Buy the best cookware you can afford, as quality pieces will last you for many years to come. This cookware will help with preparing, cooking, and storing all of the wonderful meals you will be enjoying:

heavy-bottomed stainless steel skillet, saucepan, and stockpot

nonstick skillet

heavy roasting pan

glass storage containers with lids, and baking dishes

plastic cutting boards

traditional blender and immersion blender

food processor

knives (chef's, paring, and serrated)

water filter

spice grinder

The Well-Stocked Healthy Pantry

Now that your kitchen has been purged of unhealthy stuff, the key to making delicious food easily is to always have essential ingredients on hand. I've included pantry staples as just a sample of what's out there. You will find many of these items in the recipes in this chapter as well as in the 7-Day Plan for Radiant Skin. Buy what appeals to you and your family. Try new things, experiment with new flavors, and experience food all in the name of healthy, beautiful skin. By keeping your kitchen stocked, you'll always have a quick and delicious meal at your fingertips. Even with pantry products, always try to buy organic.

Flour

rice flour

spelt flour (a whole-grain organic, unbleached flour that is a good source of fiber and B-complex vitamins, with a protein content of 10% to 25% more than other common varieties of commercial wheat flour)

unbleached whole-wheat flour

Dried Herbs and Spices

allspice

bay leaves

cardamom seeds

cinnamon

cloves

coriander

cumin

juniper berries

nutmeg (whole)

white peppercorns (black peppercorns, with their exterior shells,
are harder for the digestive system to break down)

Dried Legumes

adzuki beans

black beans

cannellini beans (all white)

chickpeas

green split peas

lentils

mung beans

Miscellaneous

bee pollen (Bee pollen contains the male gametes of plants
found as small dust pellets in the stamen of flowers. Bee pollen is
thought to help build the immune system and provide energy. It

contains 35% protein, 55% carbohydrates, 2% fatty acids, and 3% minerals and vitamins. It is high in B-complex vitamins and vitamins A, C, D, and E. It also contains lecithin, beta-carotene, and selenium. This combination of elements makes bee pollen an excellent source of antioxidants.)

Ezekiel bread or sprouted grain bread (This bread is made from whole sprouted wheat, spelt, Kamut, or other grains. Sprouted grain bread involves soaking the grain and allowing it to sprout. The sprouted seedlings are then mashed together and baked. Sprouting allows the enzymes in the grain to convert some of the carbohydrates and fats to vitamins, minerals, and amino acids. Due to the changes that take place, sprouted grain bread typically is higher in protein, fiber, and certain vitamins and minerals than regular bread. It is also less refined and processed than even stone-ground wheat bread, so it is thought to have less of an impact on blood sugar. Sprouted grain bread is available in rolls and loaves of various shapes and sizes, and it may contain a variety of grains.)

a variety of herbal teas

miso paste (Also known as fermented bean paste, it is a concentrated, savory paste made from soybeans often mixed with a grain such as rice, barley, or wheat that is fermented with a yeast mold *(koji),* then combined with salt and water. The mixture is aged from 1 month to 3 years before being sold for use in soups, dressings, marinades, dips, and other foods.)

Oils (Store in a cool, dry place)

canola oil

extra-virgin olive oil

grapeseed oil

toasted and plain sesame oil

macadamia nut oil

Onion family

garlic

leeks

onions

scallions

shallots

Rice

arborio

basmati

jasmine

short- and long-grain brown

wild

Seaweed

(Seaweed is very rich in minerals and calcium. Seaweeds are often used in soups [such as miso], salads, and as part of sushi presentations. They are usually sold in dried forms in sheets or cakes and are available at Asian specialty markets or health food stores. This list is just a sample of what's available.)

agar

arame

dulse

hijiki

nori

wakame

Seeds and Nuts

almonds

cashews

flaxseeds (These seeds are a good source of protein, fiber, vitamins, minerals, and lignins, a natural plant chemical that contains antioxidants. They are considered helpful as a gentle natural laxative as well. Ground flaxseeds can be added to a variety of cooked or raw foods. Seeds are available preground or can be ground in a spice grinder. Flaxseed oil can also be used as an alternative.)

macadamia nuts

pecans

pine nuts

pumpkin seeds

sesame seeds (white or black)

sunflower seeds

walnuts

Vinegars

apple cider

balsamic

red wine

rice

sherry

white wine

Whole Grains

amaranth

brown rice

bulgur

kasha

millet

oatmeal (whole or rolled oats)

quinoa

spelt

wild rice

In addition to the dry pantry items, shop regularly every few days for fresh organic items. Here are some for consideration.

Dairy

fresh or aged goat cheese

organic eggs

fresh or aged sheep's milk cheese

soy cheese

Fruits and Vegetables

apples

avocados

arugula

beets

berries

bok choy

broccoli

cabbage, all types

carrots

celery

celery root

fennel

garlic

kale

lemons

lettuce (all varieties including Boston, romaine, and red leaf)

limes

papaya

parsnips

pears

pineapple

spinach

turnips

vine-ripe tomatoes

winter squash, all types such as acorn, butternut, and spaghetti

yams

zucchini

Fresh Herbs and Seasonings

basil

chervil

ginger

marjoram

parsley

rosemary

tarragon

thyme

Protein

organic chicken

tempeh

tofu

organic turkey

wild (not farm-raised) fish

Getting the Healthy Goods: Shopping for Your Food

Once upon a time, the milkman delivered dairy products to your door, the corner grocer knew your name, and the butcher knew how you liked your meat cut. But for the most part, those days are over, and supermarkets and super-duper megamarts have taken over the distribution of food to the American public. In order to shop for your skin, your health, and the health of your family, you may have to do a little work to hunt down what you need. Start by seeking out as many organic products as you can find. They are worth whatever extra they may cost. Take some time to look on-line or in the phone book for what's available in your neighborhood. Most supermarket chains now have an organic produce section. Many have organic chicken and meats, and they sell wild rather than farm-raised seafood.

If your local grocer does not offer the organic products you want, look for packaged staples on-line at gourmetpantry.com, organic.com, shopnatural.com, and shopnature.com. Talk to your local grocery store manager about the possibility of carrying more organic products. The more demand, the more likely stores will take action to stock more healthful products. Also try visiting your local farmers' market for fresh produce, or finding out if your area has a Community Supported Agriculture (CSA) cooperative from which to purchase produce. Make sure that what you are buying from the farmers' market or CSA is organic.

Here are a few things you should keep in mind before you enter the grocery store:

- Don't shop when you're hungry. When you shop with an empty stomach, everything looks too good to pass up. In fact, studies have shown that people who shop hungry end up spending 17 percent more at the checkout!

- Give yourself enough time to shop. Preparing a meal begins with picking out the right foods. If you're in a hurry or not paying attention, it will show up in your meals.

- Remember that balance and variety are the keys to health, beauty, and a satisfying meal.

- Buy what's in season; it will be fresher and usually less expensive.

- Buy fresh. Rather than shopping with a set menu in mind, be flexible based on what your butcher or fishmonger has to offer.

Labels 101

In 1990, the Food and Drug Administration made it mandatory for all packaged foods to list nutritional information. You've seen the labels on the back of everything from bread to chocolate pudding, and they contain important information organized in two sections: Nutritional Facts and Ingredients. Make it your business to read these labels every time an item goes into your shopping cart. For a full description of what each element of a nutritional label indicates, check out the Food and Drug Administration's website at www.fda.gov.

Go to your kitchen and take out a packaged or canned product. The total fat listing in any product is broken down into various categories including Saturated Fat, Trans Fat, Polyunsaturated Fat, and Monounsaturated Fat. Trans fats, as discussed in chapter 1, are unsaturated or polyunsaturated fats that have been turned into saturated fats through a process called hydrogenation. This process adds hydrogen molecules to polyunsaturated oils such as soybean oil in order to make them solid or saturated fats. Avoid products with trans fats or saturated fats whenever possible.

Below the nutritional information on packaged products, the ingredients are listed in descending order according to the amount of the ingredient used. If sugar is the first ingredient on the list, it means there is more sugar than anything else in the item. Look at the ingredients label on a fruit drink. On many, you will find that actual fruit juice is rarely the first or even the second ingredient listed. Some fruit drinks contain as little as 10 percent real fruit juice. The majority of the product is often water, sugar, and artificial flavoring. And, as always, be aware of additives, chemicals, and all of the other toxins that you can ingest without even knowing it.

Hidden sugar is another ingredient you can spot if you know what to look for. Sugar is often "disguised" as fructose, corn syrup, neotame, acesulfame, sucralose, lactose, sorbitol, mannitol, xylitol, maltitol, maltose, and dextrose. Also, many low-fat foods include sugar to make up for the missing flavor when fat is taken out.

Finally, don't be swayed by the word *natural*. Just because something says "natural" on the package doesn't necessarily mean it's good for you. If the first three ingredients listed on the label are things you know you should keep away from, such as sugar, salt, or fat, no matter how natural, organic, or healthy the product is supposed to be, don't buy it. Moreover, if you review the list of ingredients and you don't know what an ingredient is, you probably shouldn't be eating it, which is why I stress again and again that cooking your own food is truly the best way to achieve beautiful skin and a healthy, well-functioning body.

The best way to avoid eating toxic foods is to stay away from as much processed food as possible. If, however, you choose to use a processed product, such as a can of beans, I urge you to buy a brand that uses organic beans and as few other added ingredients or preservatives as possible. Fresh food in its natural state is always the better alternative. If necessary, it is preferable that you use frozen organic ingredients rather than nonorganic fresh ones.

Recipes for Revitalized Skin

While I am a busy working woman with a bicoastal business, I still look forward to cooking for myself and loved ones. There is something cathartic about taking the best-quality raw ingredients and transforming them into a wonderful meal with little or no fuss. Sitting down at the end of the day to a meal is also when we can reflect and be very much "in the moment." With so much going on in everybody's lives, it's important to take time out to appreciate each other and the food on the table. It is extremely important that your body and mind be in a state of "at rest and digest," before you start to eat in order to achieve optimal digestion. Improperly digested food can turn into toxic waste in your system, which can lead to a weakened immune system and poorer health.

Although I prefer to cook and eat at home, I, of course, do eat in restaurants. In order to avoid foods that may be bad for me when I go out to eat, I tend to order simply. I start with a salad and ask for olive oil and lemon on the side, which I then drizzle over the salad. I select a lean protein (chicken breast or fish) prepared with minimal fats or sauces. Most restaurants can accommodate a request for simply grilled fish or chicken even if it doesn't appear on the menu. I then get a side of whatever vegetable appeals to me, either steamed or sautéed in a little bit of olive oil. I avoid starches, especially the bread basket. Ordering this way allows me to feel healthy and satisfied, and I know I won't have done any damage to my skin or my body.

I started making the recipes in this chapter years ago, as I needed a variety of healthy, delicious foods that could mostly be prepared in less than 30 minutes. After coming home from a day of treating clients, the last thing I wanted to do was slave over a stove for hours or make complicated recipes with dozens of steps and ingredients. These recipes are my standards. They are quick and easy, and I make them as often as possible. With the proper equipment and a stocked pantry, it's easy to throw a healthy meal together quickly.

These recipes feature a variety of foods that will benefit your skin and your overall health. Many of them are called for in the 7-Day Plan for Radiant Skin, but they can be prepared anytime for any occasion. I tend to cook with a generous amount of fresh herbs because of the major benefits they offer my skin. Feel free to add whatever amount of herbs tastes right to you. Experiment with different proteins, herbs, and spices to ultimately develop some of your own favorite recipes.

Soups

These soups contain lots of antioxidants and vitamins to help ward off free radicals and prevent skin damage. Eat them as often as possible. They can be served pureed or chunky. Choose whichever texture you most desire.

Adzuki Bean Soup

This bean, originally from Asia, is believed to be helpful as a kidney cleanser. I have found this mineral-rich soup helps get rid of dark circles and shadows under the eyes, and it alleviates bloating and water retention. Try to eat this soup at least six times a month for optimal effect. Adzuki beans can be found in your local health food store. • **Serves 6**

2 cups adzuki beans, soaked overnight in water to cover

1 tablespoon toasted sesame oil

1 small onion, chopped

1 carrot, chopped

1 stalk celery, chopped

2 teaspoons cumin

½ teaspoon turmeric

3 garlic cloves, chopped

2 tablespoons freshly grated ginger

2 quarts chicken stock *or* vegetable stock *or* water

Sea salt

freshly ground white pepper

½ cup freshly squeezed lime juice

½ cup freshly chopped cilantro

Drain the beans. Place the beans, along with 5 cups of cold water, in a large heavy-bottom pot and bring to a boil. Cook 1 hour, or until tender. Drain the beans and set aside.

In a stockpot, heat the sesame oil over medium heat. Add the onions, carrots, celery, cumin, and turmeric, and sauté until tender, about 10 minutes. Add the garlic and ginger and cook 1 minute. Add the beans and stock, and salt and pepper to taste. Simmer an additional 25 minutes or until beans are tender, stirring occasionally.

Transfer the soup to a blender in batches and puree until smooth (or use an immersion blender). Return the pureed soup to the pot and reheat. Add the lime juice and cilantro. Taste and adjust seasonings if necessary. Divide the soup among six bowls.

Tuscan Bean Soup

This fragrant, savory soup is full of antioxidants, which keep collagen strong and your skin in great shape. Serve it with Baby Spinach and Arugula Salad (page 127) and a piece of sprouted grain bread for a wonderful lunch. • **Serves 6 to 8**

2 cups dried pinto beans, white beans, or cannellini beans,
    soaked overnight in water to cover
1 bay leaf
½ teaspoon freshly ground white pepper, plus more to taste
3 garlic cloves
2 tablespoons extra-virgin olive oil
1 small onion, chopped
1 leek, thinly sliced
1 carrot, chopped
2 cups chopped kale
1 cup whole canned plum tomatoes, seeded and chopped
4 garlic cloves, thinly sliced
3 quarts chicken stock
½ cup freshly chopped flat-leaf parsley
½ cup freshly chopped basil
1 tablespoon freshly chopped rosemary
Sea salt

Drain the beans. In a large pot, bring 2 quarts water, the beans, bay leaf, ½ teaspoon white pepper, and garlic cloves to a boil. Cook 1 hour over medium heat or until tender. Drain well and discard the bay leaf.

In another large pot, heat the olive oil over medium heat. Add the onions, leeks, carrots, kale, tomatoes, and sliced garlic and cook 10 minutes or until the vegetables are tender. Add the beans, chicken stock, and salt, if desired, and cook 30 minutes.

Remove the pot from the heat and let the soup sit 15 minutes. Then add the parsley, basil, and rosemary.

Transfer the soup to a blender in batches and puree until smooth (or use an immersion blender). Return the pureed soup to the pot and reheat. Taste and adjust seasonings if necessary before serving.

Mung Bean Vegetable Soup

Mung beans are one of the most important because of their therapeutic power. It is suggested that they are good for cleansing the heart and liver and beneficial in reducing toxicity in these organs. If eaten regularly (once a week), this soup can help clear up a troubled complexion, dissipate rosacea, and help control breakouts. And best of all, it tastes delicious. • Serves 6 to 8

2 cups dried mung beans, soaked overnight in water to cover

2 tablespoons extra-virgin olive oil

1 small onion, chopped

1 bunch scallions, thinly sliced

1 carrot, chopped

3 garlic cloves, thinly sliced

3 quarts chicken stock *or* vegetable stock *or* water

1 cup cooked brown rice

Freshly ground nutmeg

Sea salt

Freshly ground white pepper

½ cup freshly chopped flat-leaf parsley

½ cup freshly chopped basil

Drain the beans. Place the beans, along with 5 cups cold water, in a large pot, cover, and bring to a low boil. Cook 1 hour or until tender. Drain the beans and set aside.

In a soup pot, heat the olive oil over medium heat. Add the onions, scallions, and carrots and sauté until translucent, about 10 minutes. Add the garlic and cook 1 minute. Add the beans and chicken stock and cook about 30 minutes. Add the rice and season with nutmeg, salt, and pepper to taste. Add additional stock if the soup gets too thick.

Just before serving, add the parsley and basil. Taste and adjust seasonings if necessary.

Creamy Broccoli Soup

This soup is full of antioxidants, vitamin C, and iron, which are needed to maintain a healthy immune system and beautiful skin. Broccoli is a cruciferous vegetable and is thought to help slow or possibly prevent the development of cancer. Children who don't normally like eating vegetables really enjoy this flavorful soup. • *Serves 6 to 8*

1 tablespoon extra-virgin olive oil
1 pound broccoli, chopped into small pieces
1 large onion, diced
1 carrot, diced
2 stalks celery, chopped
2 garlic cloves, chopped
1 cup chopped kale
2 quarts chicken stock
½ teaspoon freshly ground nutmeg
Sea salt
Freshly ground white pepper
½ cup freshly chopped flat-leaf parsley
½ cup freshly chopped basil or tarragon

In a large skillet heat the olive oil over medium heat. Add the broccoli, onions, carrots, celery, garlic, and kale. Sauté about 10 minutes.

Transfer the vegetables to a large stock pot along with the chicken stock. Bring to a boil over high heat, then reduce heat to a simmer. Add the nutmeg, salt, and pepper to taste. Simmer 20 minutes. Garnish with parsley and basil and serve.

Transfer the soup to a blender in batches and puree until smooth (or use an immersion blender). Return the pureed soup to the pot and reheat. Taste and adjust seasonings if necessary before serving.

Chickpea and Roasted Garlic Soup

This hearty soup is thick and wonderfully rich. Chickpeas help the digestive system, which in turn helps clear up complexion problems. The garlic is sweet from the roasting and a good boost for your immune system. • *Serves 6 to 8*

2 tablespoons extra-virgin olive oil

1 small onion, chopped

1 carrot, chopped

1 stalk celery, chopped

2 cups cooked chickpeas

1 large head roasted garlic (page 185)

2 teaspoons freshly chopped rosemary

2 quarts chicken stock

Sea salt

Freshly ground white pepper

Juice and zest from 1 lemon

½ cup freshly chopped flat-leaf parsley

In a soup pot, heat the olive oil over medium heat. Add the onions, carrots, and celery and sauté 10 minutes. Add the chickpeas, roasted garlic, rosemary, and chicken stock. Cook 20 minutes.

Transfer the soup to a blender in batches and puree until smooth (or use an immersion blender). Return the pureed soup to the pot and reheat. Taste and adjust seasonings. Just before serving, add the lemon juice, lemon zest, and parsley and stir to combine.

Roasted Butternut Squash Soup

Butternut, as well as all winter squashes, is an excellent source of beta-carotene, which is an essential immune booster. Warm and comforting, this soup is a perfect starter for a cold-weather dinner party. • **Serves 4 to 6**

1 large butternut squash, halved and seeded
1 tablespoon extra-virgin olive oil
1 large onion, chopped
1 garlic clove, chopped
3 quarts chicken stock
Freshly ground nutmeg
Sea salt
Freshly ground white pepper
3 tablespoons freshly chopped basil *or* tarragon

Preheat the oven to 375 degrees F.

Place the squash cut side up in a roasting pan and roast, covered, 30 minutes, or until tender when pierced with a fork. Remove from the oven and allow to cool. When cooled, peel the squash and cut it into small chunks. Set aside.

In a large stockpot, heat the olive oil over medium heat. Add the onions and garlic and sauté until translucent, about 5 minutes. Add the roasted squash and chicken stock. Add the nutmeg, salt, and pepper to taste and cook 30 minutes.

Transfer the soup to a blender in batches and puree until smooth (or use an immersion blender). Return the pureed soup to the pot and reheat. Taste and adjust seasonings if necessary.

Ladle the soup into serving bowls and sprinkle with basil or tarragon and another grating of nutmeg before serving.

Miso Soup

Soy paste miso is high in protein, B vitamins, and isoflavones (plant estrogens), and it is thought to contain enzymes that stimulate digestion. You can find the ingredients for this traditional Japanese soup at many supermarkets or at on-line Asian grocers. For an Asian-inspired dinner, serve with Asian Roasted Chicken (page 132) and Ginger-Steamed Baby Bok Choy (page 172). • *Serves 4*

    6-inch kombu leaf
    3 tablespoons miso paste
    2 tablespoons bonito flakes
    1 cup cubed firm tofu
    1 teaspoon toasted sesame seeds
    3 tablespoons thinly sliced scallions

Rinse the kombu leaf and blot the salt off with a damp paper towel. Place the kombu leaf in a stock pot. Add 3 cups water and bring to a boil over high heat. Cover and reduce heat to low. Cook 20 minutes. Remove the kombu from the pot with a slotted spoon and discard.

Place the miso paste in a small bowl. Add 2 to 3 tablespoons of the kombu cooking liquid and stir to a creamy consistency.

Add the miso paste, bonito flakes, tofu, and sesame seeds to the pot of cooking liquid. Cover, remove from heat, and let sit 10 minutes.

Evenly distribute the scallions in the bottom of four serving bowls. Pour the miso broth over the scallions and serve.

Salads

There is no end to the health benefits of eating fresh salads at least once if not twice a day. The fiber, minerals, vitamins, and trace elements help keep your digestive system balanced and healthy. An unhealthy digestive system is a precursor to a number of diseases such as cancer, arthritis, and high blood pressure. The vitamins and minerals found in raw vegetables deliver valuable nutrients to your skin. Salads also help to curb your appetite since they can be very filling. Remember to chew your raw food very well for proper absorption and elimination.

Antioxidant Salad

This salad is filled with fiber and antioxidant-rich vegetables that will help keep your skin looking fresh and young. It is offered for lunch and dinner throughout the 7-Day Plan for Radiant Skin (page 59). • **Serves 6**

1 head romaine lettuce, torn into pieces

1 small bunch arugula, torn into pieces

½ cup freshly chopped flat-leaf parsely

6 freshly chopped basil leaves

1 carrot, thinly sliced

1 stalk celery, thinly sliced

¼ cup radish sprouts

1 fennel bulb, thinly sliced

1 teaspoon toasted sesame seeds *or* 1 teaspoon ground
flaxseeds *or* ¼ cup toasted pumpkin seeds

Lemon-Lime Olive Oil Dressing (page 177) *or* Sesame-Ginger
Carrot Dressing (page 179)

Combine all ingredients except the dressing in a large bowl. Toss with just enough dressing to lightly coat. Serve immediately.

Cleansing Salad

Eating plenty of salads is crucial to a healthy colon. This salad is loaded with the vitamins and nutrients that help minimize your pores and make your skin more radiant. It is offered as part of the 7-Day Plan for Radiant Skin (page 59). • **Serves 6 to 8**

> 1 head chicory, torn into pieces
> 1 head radicchio, torn into pieces
> 1 vine-ripened tomato, thinly sliced
> ½ seedless hot house cucumber, thinly sliced
> 1 stalk celery, thinly sliced
> ½ cup freshly chopped flat-leaf parsley *or* tarragon
> ¼ cup freshly chopped basil
> 1 teaspoon toasted sesame seeds *or* 1 teaspoon ground
>   flaxseeds *or* ¼ cup toasted pumpkin seeds
> Lemon-Lime Olive Oil Dressing (page 177) *or* Sherry Vinaigrette
>   (page 178)

Combine all ingredients except the dressing in a large chilled bowl. Toss with just enough dressing to lightly coat. Serve immediately.

Watercress Salad with Pine Nuts and Roasted Shallots

This is an elegant salad to serve as a first course. Aside from its wonderful peppery taste, watercress contains beneficial antioxidants and is a good source of vitamins E and C, which help prevent signs of aging. • **Serves 4**

4 shallots, halved
2 tablespoons extra-virgin olive oil
¼ teaspoon sea salt
¼ teaspoon freshly ground white pepper
1 bunch watercress
½ cup freshly chopped flat-leaf parsley
3 tablespoons freshly chopped basil *or* tarragon
½ cup toasted pine nuts *or* toasted chopped walnuts
Sherry Vinaigrette (page 178)

Preheat the oven to 350 degrees F.

Place the shallots in a small baking dish and drizzle with the olive oil. Add the salt and pepper to taste and combine until the shallots are well coated. Roast for 30 minutes or until tender. Remove from the oven and allow to cool.

Combine the shallots with the watercress, parsley, basil or tarragon, and pine nuts or walnuts in a chilled bowl and toss with just enough vinaigrette to lightly coat. Serve immediately.

Beet and Goat Cheese Salad

I often serve this beautifully plated salad at dinner parties. I find it indulgent because of the rich, tangy, nutty flavor of the goat cheese—a good choice for calcium and protein. • **Serves 4**

   4 beets, trimmed
   1 tablespoon plus 1 teaspoon extra-virgin olive oil
   1 red onion, thinly sliced
   3 tablespoons freshly chopped basil
   4 ounces goat cheese, crumbled
   Sherry Vinaigrette (page 178)
   Sea salt
   Freshly ground white pepper

Preheat the oven to 400 degrees F.

Place the beets in a small baking dish and fill with one-quarter inch of water. Drizzle 1 tablespoon of olive oil over the top. Cover with aluminum foil and roast the beets for 1 hour. Allow to cool and slip the skins off with a paper towel. Slice the beets approximately one-eighth inch thick and set aside.

Meanwhile, heat 1 teaspoon of olive oil in a small skillet over medium heat. Add the onions and sauté until translucent, about 10 minutes. Remove from the heat and let cool.

Arrange the beet slices on four serving plates or a large platter. Sprinkle the beets with the basil and goat cheese. Drizzle the vinaigrette evenly over the beets. Add salt and pepper to taste and serve.

Fennel and Red Cabbage Salad

*In Italy, fennel is considered a digestive aid and is often eaten after a meal.
Enjoy the licorice-like taste and crunchy texture of fennel in a salad or by
itself, sliced and dipped in olive oil.* • **Serves 4 to 6**

1 large head fennel, thinly sliced
1 small head red cabbage, thinly sliced
4 tablespoons freshly chopped basil
½ cup toasted chopped pecans *or* walnuts
½ cup crumbled feta cheese
Sea salt
Freshly ground white pepper
Lemon-Lime Olive Oil Dressing (page 177)

Combine all ingredients except the dressing in a chilled bowl. Toss with
just enough dressing to lightly coat. Serve immediately.

Baby Spinach and Arugula Salad

This combination of dark leafy greens, both subtle and spicy, offers an iron boost for your blood that will benefit your skin as well. Serve this simple salad as an accompaniment to Herb-Roasted Chicken (page 130). • *Serves 4 to 6*

½ pound baby spinach
1 bunch baby arugula
1 stalk celery, thinly sliced
1 carrot, thinly sliced
¼ cup freshly chopped flat-leaf parsley
¼ cup freshly chopped basil *or* tarragon
Sea salt
Freshly ground white pepper
Sherry Vinaigrette (page 178)

Combine all ingredients except the dressing in a chilled bowl. Toss with just enough dressing to lightly coat. Serve immediately.

Grilled Zucchini and Asparagus Salad

This delicious salad is full of vitamin C and other antioxidants to keep your skin clear and your collagen strong. This is a great side dish for grilled meat. I prefer stovetop grilling rather than gas or charcoal grilling to avoid the possibility of toxins being absorbed by the food. • **Serves 4 to 6**

2 tablespoons extra-virgin olive oil

1 tablespoon balsamic vinegar

1 teaspoon sea salt

Freshly ground white pepper to taste

1½ pounds zucchini, peeled and sliced lengthwise ⅛ inch thick

1 pound asparagus, trimmed

¼ cup freshly chopped flat-leaf parsley

¼ cup freshly chopped basil

4 ounces goat cheese *or* feta cheese, crumbled

Zest and juice from 1 lemon

Preheat a grill pan on the stove 1 to 2 minutes.

Combine the olive oil, vinegar, sea salt, and pepper in a bowl. Brush the zucchini and asparagus with the vinaigrette. Grill the vegetables in the preheated pan for a few minutes on each side until slightly brown.

Transfer the vegetables to a serving dish. Sprinkle with the parsley, basil, goat cheese or feta cheese, lemon zest, and lemon juice. Taste and adjust seasonings if necessary before serving.

Chicken, Turkey, Fish, and Tofu

Low-fat protein is crucial for keeping skin strong and firm and for helping to prevent premature aging. Be sure to eat 3 to 4 ounces of protein at lunch and dinner every day.

Herb-Roasted Chicken

I find that chicken, along with organic vegetables and healthy fats such as extra-virgin olive oil, helps protect the skin from drying out. Serve with Quinoa Pilaf (page 164) and Brocolli with Garlic (page 170). • **Serves 4 to 6**

3- to 4-pound organic chicken

1 to 2 teaspoons kosher salt

Freshly ground white pepper

Juice and zest from 1 lemon

3 tablespoons extra-virgin olive oil

½ cup freshly chopped flat-leaf parsley

1 tablespoon fresh thyme

1 tablespoon chopped rosemary

1 bay leaf

3 garlic cloves, thinly sliced

1 stalk celery, chopped

1 onion, thinly sliced

1 leek, thinly sliced

½ cup dry white wine

Place a pan of water on the bottom rack of the oven to prevent the chicken from drying out.

Preheat the oven to 375 degrees F.

Lightly oil a roasting pan. Wash the chicken in a pot with cold water and the kosher salt. Rinse and dry with paper towels. Rub 1 teaspoon each of salt and pepper inside the cavity of the chicken. Rub the lemon juice, lemon zest, and olive oil inside the cavity and on the outside of the chicken.

Place as much of the parsley, thyme, rosemary, bay leaf, garlic, celery, onions, and leeks in the cavity of the chicken as possible. Whatever doesn't fit should be placed on the bottom of the prepared pan to create a bed for the chicken to sit on. Place the chicken on the vegetable bed and pour the white wine over it. Sprinkle salt and pepper in the bottom of the pan around the chicken.

Roast the chicken on the middle rack of the oven. After 30 minutes, start basting the chicken with the pan juices every 20 minutes or so for 1 hour. Insert an instant-read thermometer to test for doneness. It should register 175 degrees F in the thigh and 170 degrees F in the breast. After the chicken is done, cover it with aluminum foil and let sit at least 15 minutes before carving.

Asian Roasted Chicken

*For a perfect meal, serve this delicious dish with Wild Rice Salad (page 163)
and Ginger-Steamed Baby Bok Choy (page 172).* • **Serves 4 to 5**

3- to 4-pound organic chicken
1 to 2 teaspoons kosher salt
Freshly ground white pepper
1½ tablespoons extra-virgin olive oil
1½ tablespoons toasted sesame oil
½ cup sliced scallions
½ cup freshly chopped cilantro
1 tablespoon tamari *or* low-sodium soy sauce
1 tablespoon rice wine vinegar
2 tablespoons minced garlic
1 tablespoon freshly grated ginger
Juice and zest from 1 lime
6 shallots

Wash the chicken in a pot with cold water and the kosher salt. Rinse and
dry with paper towels. Rub 1 teaspoon each of salt and pepper inside the
cavity of the chicken. Place the chicken in a deep bowl.

To make a marinade, combine the olive oil, sesame oil, scallions, cilantro,
tamari or soy sauce, rice wine vinegar, garlic, ginger, lime juice, and lime
zest in a small bowl.

Pour the marinade inside and all over the outside of the chicken. Cover
with plastic wrap and place in the refrigerator a minimum of 3 hours.

Place a pan of water on the bottom rack of the oven to prevent the
chicken from drying out.

Preheat the oven to 375 degrees F.

Lightly oil a roasting pan. Remove the chicken from the refrigerator and pat the outside of the chicken dry with paper towels. Rub the skin with the remaining olive oil and reseason with salt and pepper. Place the chicken in the prepared roasting pan. Place the shallots around the chicken.

Roast the chicken on the middle rack of the oven. After 30 minutes, start basting the chicken with the pan juices every 20 minutes or so for 1 hour. Insert an instant-read thermometer to test for doneness. It should register 175 degrees F in the thigh and 170 degrees F in the breast. After the chicken is done, turn off the oven, cover the chicken with aluminum foil, and let sit at least 15 minutes before carving.

Tuscan Chicken with Rosemary and Plum Tomatoes

This dish is quick, easy to make, and has great flavor. This is a great meal for the whole family or for entertaining. Serve with Fava Beans (page 157), and Cleansing Salad (page 123). • **Serves 4 to 6**

3- to 4-pound organic chicken, cut into 8 to 10 pieces, skin
   removed
Kosher salt
Freshly ground white pepper
2 tablespoons extra-virgin olive oil
1 cup chopped onions
1 cup whole canned plum tomatoes, seeded and chopped
6 garlic cloves, thinly sliced
2 tablespoons freshly chopped rosemary
1 teaspoon freshly chopped thyme
Juice and zest from 1 lemon

Preheat the oven to 375 degrees F.

Wash the chicken pieces in a pot with cold water and the kosher salt. Rinse and dry with paper towels. Season with salt and pepper to taste.

In a large ovenproof skillet, heat the olive oil over medium heat. Cook the chicken in batches until it is nicely browned, about 5 to 7 minutes on each side. Remove the chicken from the pan and set aside.

To the same pan add the onions, tomatoes, garlic, rosemary, and thyme and sauté for 5 minutes. Add the lemon juice and salt and pepper to taste. Scrape down the bottom of the pan to extract flavor from the renderings left behind by the chicken. Simmer on low heat for

10 minutes until the mixture has thickened slightly. Return the chicken to the pan.

Transfer the skillet to the oven and bake, covered, 30 to 45 minutes or until juices at the thigh joint run clean. Remove from the oven and let rest 10 minutes. Add the lemon zest just before serving.

Chicken Okra Stew

This thick, rich stew is a wonderful comfort food. Okra contains lots of vitamin C, which has been found to help reduce the risk of heart disease. It is also full of osteoporosis-fighting nutrients including calcium, potassium, magnesium, and beta-carotene. Serve this stew along with Antioxidant Salad (page 122) and Mashed Celery Root (page 169). • *Serves 4 to 6*

3- to 4-pound organic chicken, cut into 8 to 10 pieces, skin removed
Kosher salt
Sea salt
Freshly ground white pepper
2 tablespoons extra-virgin olive oil
1 onion, finely chopped
1 teaspoon turmeric
2 green chilies, seeded and chopped
1 pound small okra, thinly sliced
3 vine-ripened tomatoes, cored and chopped
4 garlic cloves, finely chopped
Juice and zest from 2 limes
1 cup freshly chopped cilantro

Preheat the oven to 375 degrees F.

Place a pan of water on the bottom rack of the oven to prevent the chicken from drying out.

Wash the chicken pieces in a pot with cold water and the kosher salt. Rinse and dry with paper towels. Season with sea salt and pepper to taste.

In a large skillet, heat the olive oil over medium heat. Cook the chicken in batches until it is nicely browned on all sides, about 5 to 7 minutes on each side. Remove the chicken from the pan and set aside.

Reduce the heat to low and add the onions and turmeric to the pan. Sauté until the onions are translucent, about 5 minutes. Add the chilies, okra, tomatoes, and garlic and continue sautéing until the tomato breaks down and the okra releases its gelatinous quality.

Transfer the chicken and any juices that have accumulated back to the pan. Add the lime juice. Transfer to the oven and bake 45 minutes or until an instant-read thermometer registers 170 degrees F.

Remove from the oven and stir in the lime zest and cilantro. Taste and adjust seasonings if necessary. Let sit 15 minutes before serving.

Roast Turkey

This classic recipe is easy to prepare. I make this wonderful turkey every year for Thanksgiving, and I also use the same preparation throughout the year when I make a turkey breast. The leftovers are great in a salad or on a slice of sprouted grain bread covered with Roasted Garlic Spread (page 185) or White Bean Dip (page 180). • **Serves 10 to 12**

12- to 15-pound organic turkey
Kosher salt
3 tablespoons extra-virgin olive oil
2 large onions, chopped
3 stalks celery, chopped
1 leek, sliced
2 tablespoons freshly chopped rosemary
3 freshly chopped sage leaves
1 teaspoon freshly chopped thyme
Freshly ground white pepper
4 garlic cloves, chopped
1 red onion, chopped
8 shallots
Juice and zest from 1 lemon
2 to 3 cups chicken stock *or* vegetable stock *or* water

Place a pan of water on the bottom rack of the oven to prevent the turkey from drying out.

Preheat the oven to 350 degrees F.

Wash the turkey in a pot with cold water and the kosher salt. Rinse and dry with paper towels.

In a large skillet, heat 2 tablespoons of the olive oil over medium heat. Add the onions, celery, leeks, rosemary, sage, and thyme. Season with salt and pepper to taste. Cook until the onions are translucent, about 10 minutes.

Add the garlic and cook 1 minute. Remove from the heat and let the mixture cool.

Rub the inside and outside of the turkey with the remaining tablespoon of olive oil. Rub inside the cavity and around the outside with salt and pepper. Insert the vegetable mixture inside the cavity.

Place the prepared turkey in a large roasting pan and scatter the red onion and shallots around the turkey. Pour lemon juice over the top of the turkey. Season with salt and pepper to taste. Add 1 cup chicken stock, vegetable stock, or water to the pan.

Bake 15 minutes per pound (a 12-pound turkey would take 3 hours). Add the remaining stock or water throughout roasting to keep liquid in the pan. After the skin turns golden brown, sprinkle with the lemon zest. Then lightly grease a large piece of aluminum foil and place over the turkey. Baste the turkey every 20 minutes until done. Insert an instant-read thermometer to test for doneness. It should register 180 degrees F in the thigh and 170 degrees F in the breast.

Remove the turkey from the oven and let sit at least 15 minutes before carving.

Vegetable-Stuffed Turkey Breast

While this dish looks as if you might have slaved over it, it's actually quite easy to prepare. I like to serve it when I entertain because of the wonderful presentation the vegetable-stuffed breast offers. Serve with Roasted Cauliflower (page 171). • *Serves 8*

4- to 5-pound organic turkey breast, butterflied with skin on
    (you can ask your butcher to do this) and pounded flat
Sea salt
Freshly ground white pepper
2 tablespoons extra-virgin olive oil
1 large onion, finely chopped
2 stalks celery, chopped
1 cup chopped kale
1 leek, thinly sliced
1 small zucchini, finely chopped
1 tablespoon freshly chopped sage
1 tablespoon freshly chopped rosemary
4 garlic cloves, chopped
½ teaspoon freshly ground nutmeg
Juice and zest from 2 lemons
1 cup white wine

Place a pan of water on the bottom rack of the oven to prevent the turkey from drying out.

Preheat the oven to 375 degrees F.

Season the turkey on both sides with salt and pepper and set aside.

In a large nonstick skillet, heat 1 tablespoon of the olive oil over medium heat. Add the onions, celery, kale, leeks, zucchini, sage, and rosemary and sauté 5 minutes or until tender. Add the garlic and cook 1 minute. Add the nutmeg and salt and pepper to taste. Pour the mixture into a separate bowl and let cool.

Add the lemon juice and white wine to the pan, cook over high heat and reduce by half. Use a wooden spoon to scrape up any browned bits. Remove the reduction from the heat and set aside.

Spread the cooled mixture on top of the turkey breast and roll. Tie the breast crosswise in several places with butcher twine to secure all of the stuffing.

In a separate large skillet, heat the remaining olive oil over medium-high heat. Add the stuffed turkey breast and cook about 5 minutes on each side until browned on all sides.

Transfer the turkey breast to a roasting pan and add the white wine reduction to the bottom. Pour the reduced sauce on top. Sprinkle with the lemon zest. Add a pinch more sea salt and pepper. Cover the pan with aluminum foil and roast for 45 minutes. Remove the foil and roast for an additional 15 to 30 minutes. Insert an instant-read thermometer to test for doneness. It should register 170 degrees F.

Remove the turkey breast from the oven and let rest, covered, at least 15 minutes. Drizzle the pan juices over the turkey when ready to serve.

Sautéed Salmon with Tomato and Basil

Salmon is high in omega-3 fatty acids, which are good for the heart and may even help protect against rheumatoid arthritis and other illnesses. Be sure to ask your fishmonger if the salmon you are buying is wild, as opposed to farm-raised, which can contain dangerous levels of the chemical PCB (polychlorinated biphenyl), a toxin that the Environmental Protection Agency calls a "probable human carcinogen." Arctic char is also a wonderful substitute for the salmon dishes in this book. • *Serves 4*

2 tablespoons extra-virgin olive oil
Four 4-ounce pieces wild salmon, skin left intact
Kosher salt
Freshly ground white pepper
2 shallots, minced
¼ cup diced, seeded tomato
2 garlic cloves, thinly sliced
4 freshly chopped basil leaves
³/₄ cup white wine
Juice and zest from 1 lime

Heat a nonstick skillet over high heat. Add 1 tablespoon of the olive oil to coat the pan evenly.

Season the salmon on both sides with salt and pepper. Place the fish flesh side down in the skillet and cook 4 minutes or until golden. Turn and cook an additional 3 minutes. Transfer the fish to a heated dish.

Add the remaining olive oil to the skillet and heat over medium heat. Add the shallots, tomato, and garlic, and sauté 5 minutes. Add the white wine and reduce by half. Add the lime juice and zest and heat through.

Divide the fish among four plates, pour the sauce over the top, add basil, and serve immediately.

Wild Poached Salmon

Salmon is the best fish you can eat for your health and skin because of the fatty acids it contains. This dish can be served warm, cold, or at room temperature. It is perfect for a luncheon served alongside Brown Rice Risotto (page 162), Sautéed Brussels Sprouts (page 173), and Cleansing Salad (page 123). • **Serves 4**

1 quart vegetable stock *or* water
1 herb bundle (1 bay leaf, 1 sprig parsley, 1 sprig tarragon,
    1 sprig rosemary, and 1 sprig thyme wrapped in
    cheesecloth)
1 large shallot, finely chopped
1 tablespoon pink peppercorns, lightly crushed
Four 4-ounce pieces wild salmon
Sea salt
Freshly ground white pepper
Lemon slices

To prepare the poaching liquid, in a deep skillet combine the vegetable stock or water, herb bundle, shallots, and peppercorns and cook over medium heat.

Season both sides of the salmon with salt and pepper. When the poaching liquid is close to boiling, place the salmon in the skillet, cover, and lower heat to medium and simmer 6 minutes.

Using a slotted spoon, transfer the salmon to a serving dish and garnish with the lemon slices.

Red Snapper with Shallot-Herb Sauce

*Red snapper is a delicious fish and is available year-round. It is light and delicate and only needs a simple preparation. If you prefer, you can substitute wild grouper or striped bass for the red snapper. Serve with Ginger-Steamed Baby Bok Choy (page 172) and Wild Rice Salad (page 163). • **Serves 4***

2 tablespoons extra-virgin olive oil

Four 4-ounce pieces red snapper, skin left intact

Kosher salt

Freshly ground white pepper

2 shallots, minced

2 garlic cloves, thinly sliced

¼ cup dry white wine

Juice from 1 lemon

½ cup freshly chopped flat-leaf parsley *or* 1 tablespoon freshly chopped thyme

1 tablespoon lemon zest

Preheat a nonstick skillet for 1 minute over medium-high heat. Add the olive oil to coat the pan evenly.

Season the red snapper with salt and pepper on both sides.

Place the fish flesh side down in the skillet and cook 4 minutes or until golden. Turn and sear the skin side of the fish an additional 4 minutes. Transfer the fish from the pan and place on a heated dish.

Add the shallots and garlic to the pan and sauté 1 minute. Add the white wine and lemon juice and cook over high heat until the liquid is reduced by half. Scrape up any browned bits with a wooden spoon. Add the parsley or thyme and stir until combined.

Spoon the sauce over the fish and sprinkle with the lemon zest. Serve immediately.

Lemon-Rosemary Grilled Shrimp

This dish makes a perfect entrée or appetizer. It is versatile enough to serve at a dinner party or a backyard barbecue. You can also serve these shrimp over Antioxidant Salad (page 122) or Cleansing Salad (page 123). • ***Serves 3 to 4***

1 pound large shrimp, peeled and deveined
2 tablespoons extra-virgin olive oil
1 garlic clove, thinly sliced
1 tablespoon and 1 teaspoon freshly chopped rosemary
Sea salt
Freshly ground white pepper
Juice and zest from 1 lemon

In a large bowl, combine the shrimp, 1 tablespoon of the olive oil, garlic, 1 tablespoon of the rosemary, salt and pepper to taste, and half the lemon zest. Mix to coat.

Preheat a grill pan for 1 minute on medium-high heat.

Place the shrimp in the pan and sear 1 minute on each side. Remove the shrimp from the heat and drizzle with the remaining olive oil and lemon juice. Sprinkle with the remaining rosemary and remaining lemon zest. Serve immediately.

Asian Grilled Tuna

Tuna is a great, lean protein. The combination of these Asian influenced ingredients results in a tangy but light sauce that goes well with the tuna. Make sure to ask your fishmonger for sushi grade tuna for this recipe. Serve with Ginger-Steamed Baby Bok Choy (page 172) and Baby Spinach and Arugula Salad (page 127) with Sesame-Ginger Carrot Dressing (page 179). • *Serves 4*

Four 4-ounce pieces sushi-grade tuna
2 tablespoons toasted sesame oil
1 garlic clove, thinly sliced
2 tablespoons freshly grated ginger
1 tablespoon low-sodium soy sauce
1 tablespoon rice wine vinegar
Juice and zest from 1 lime
2 tablespoons freshly chopped cilantro
2 teaspoons toasted sesame seeds

Preheat a grill pan for 1 minute over high heat.

Brush the tuna with 1 tablespoon of the sesame oil on both sides. Place the tuna in the pan and sear 2 minutes on each side.

Transfer the tuna to a heated platter. Reduce the heat to medium. To the same pan add the remaining sesame oil, garlic, and ginger and sauté 1 minute. Add the soy sauce, rice wine vinegar, lime juice, and cook for 1 minute.

Pour the sauce over the fish and garnish with cilantro, sesame seeds, and lime zest. Serve immediately.

Seared Sea Scallops

Scallops are a wonderful source of protein, full of flavor, and low in fat. I prefer large sea scallops (as opposed to the smaller bay scallops). The texture of the scallops should be firm and they should smell fresh. Scallops should not be stored in water or a preserving brine because they will retain the water and/or brine and lose nutritional benefits and flavor. Instead, look to buy chemical-free dry-packed sea scallops. Serve with Lentilles du Puy (page 158) and Watercress Salad with Pine Nuts and Roasted Shallots (page 124). • Serves 4

1 pound sea scallops

1 teaspoon toasted sesame oil

Sea salt

Freshly ground white pepper

1 tablespoon extra-virgin olive oil

3 garlic cloves, thinly sliced

2 tablespoons freshly grated ginger

½ cup rice wine vinegar

Juice and zest from one lime

2 scallions, thinly sliced

½ cup freshly chopped cilantro

1 teaspoon toasted sesame seeds

Rinse the scallops in cold water and pat dry with paper towels.

Preheat a large, nonstick pan for 1 minute over medium-high heat.

Season the scallops with salt and pepper on both sides. Add the sesame oil to the preheated pan. Place the scallops in the preheated pan. Sauté 3 minutes on each side or until browned. Transfer the scallops to a preheated dish.

Add the olive oil, garlic, and ginger to the pan and sauté 1 minute. Add the rice wine vinegar and lime juice to the pan, scraping up any browned bits with a wooden spoon. Add the scallions and sauté 1 minute. Return the scallops to the pan and heat through.

Transfer the scallops to a serving platter. Pour the pan juices over them. Sprinkle with the cilantro, sesame seeds, and lime zest. Serve immediately.

Wild Salmon Burgers

Salmon is a wonderful source of protein, calcium, iron, omega fatty acids, and vitamins, helping to combat free radicals as well as wrinkles. Other cold-water fish containing many of these same beneficial elements include herring, snapper, and bass. Always buy wild salmon, not farm-raised, which can contain chemicals. Serve these salmon burgers on sprouted grain rolls with Roasted Garlic Spread (page 185) and whole-grain mustard on the side. • *Serves 4*

1 pound wild salmon, skin removed, finely chopped

1 tablespoon freshly grated ginger

1 garlic clove, finely chopped

½ teaspoon sea salt

Freshly grated white pepper

1 tablespoon freshly chopped cilantro

1 organic egg white, beaten

1 tablespoon toasted sesame seeds

2 teaspoons toasted sesame oil

In a large bowl combine all of the ingredients except 1 teaspoon of the sesame oil. Form the mixture into four patties. Brush the patties with the remaining sesame oil. Chill 30 minutes or more until firm.

Preheat a grill pan for 1 minute or preheat a nonstick skillet for 30 seconds over high heat. Add the burgers and sauté 3 minutes on each side or until they are opaque and cooked through.

Pan-Roasted Monkfish with Miso Sauce

This Asian-inspired dish combines the savory flavors of ginger, miso, soy sauce, and sesame oil with the delicate flavor of monkfish. This unique fish's firm flesh, similar to that of a lobster tail, accommodates the flavors well. Serve with Sautéed Brussels Sprouts (page 173) and Watercress Salad with Pine Nuts and Roasted Shallots (page 124). • ***Serves 4***

2 garlic cloves, finely chopped

2 tablespoons freshly grated ginger

1/2 cup thinly sliced scallions

1/4 cup freshly chopped cilantro

3 tablespoons miso paste

2 teaspoons soy sauce

2 tablespoons toasted sesame oil

2 tablespoons rice wine vinegar

Four 6-ounce pieces monkfish

1/4 cup freshly chopped cilantro

1/4 cup toasted sesame seeds

Juice and zest from 1 lime

To prepare the marinade, in a large bowl whisk together the garlic, ginger, scallions, cilantro, miso paste, soy sauce, sesame oil, and rice wine vinegar. Add the fish and coat with the marinade. Cover and marinate 6 hours or overnight in the refrigerator.

Preheat the oven to 400 degrees F.

Remove the fish from the marinade and place in a baking dish. Bake 10 minutes on each side. Transfer to a serving platter. Sprinkle with the cilantro, sesame seeds, lime juice, and lime zest and serve.

Grilled Tofu

Tofu, also known as soybean curd, can be found in most supermarket produce sections. Firm tofu is dense and solid and holds up well in stir-fry dishes, soups, or on the grill. Tofu is a good source of protein, B vitamins, and iron and contains no animal fat. Try eating tofu at least once a week. Just change the seasoning to add variety. Instead of turmeric, try ginger or cumin. Serve with Black Beans with Ginger and Cilantro (page 161) and Cleansing Salad (page 123). • *Serves 4*

1 teaspoon toasted sesame oil

1 teaspoon turmeric

1 garlic clove, minced

Sea salt

Freshly ground white pepper

1 pound firm tofu, sliced into four pieces

Combine the sesame oil, turmeric, garlic, and salt and pepper to taste in a bowl. Add the tofu and mix to coat. Let the tofu marinate 30 minutes or overnight in the refrigerator.

Preheat a grill pan for 1 minute over medium-high heat. Add the tofu to the pan and turn after 3 minutes. Grill 2 minutes on the other side. Serve immediately.

Tofu Casserole

This is an excellent recipe inspired by the flavors of the south of France. This dish can be served for breakfast, lunch, or dinner, and it is wonderful heated up the next day. In addition to the great taste, adding soy products such as tofu to your diet can help clear up breakouts due to hormonal imbalances caused by eating too much red meat. • *Serves 6 to 8*

2 tablespoons extra-virgin olive oil

1 large onion, finely chopped

1 carrot, finely chopped

1 stalk celery, finely chopped

½ cup freshly chopped flat-leaf parsley

½ cup freshly chopped basil

2 tablespoons freshly chopped thyme

2 tablespoons chopped Niçoise olives

1 cup whole canned plum tomatoes, seeded and chopped

2 tablespoons chopped garlic

2 pounds firm tofu, pureed in a food processor

Sea salt

Freshly ground white pepper

Preheat the oven to 350 degrees F.

Lightly grease an 8-by-10-inch baking dish with olive oil. In a nonstick skillet, heat the olive oil over medium heat. Add the onions, carrots, and celery and sauté until tender, about 10 minutes. Add the parsley, basil, thyme, and olives and sauté 2 to 3 minutes. Stir in the tomatoes, garlic, and tofu. Season with salt and pepper to taste. Remove from the heat and allow to cool.

Shape the cooled tofu mixture into a mound or loaf and transfer it to the prepared baking dish. Place the baking dish inside a larger roasting pan and fill the roasting pan with water until it comes halfway up the sides of the baking dish. Bake 30 minutes or until golden brown.

Eggplant Tofu Roliatini

Eggplant is high in vitamin C, and tofu is a great protein that is easy to digest. This recipe is for Italian food lovers who want to limit their dairy intake. Tofu is used in place of traditional ricotta cheese. You can also try substituting zucchini for the eggplant. Serve with Antioxidant Salad (page 122). • **Serves 6 to 8**

2 pounds small eggplants thinly sliced lengthwise

6 tablespoons extra-virgin olive oil

Sea salt

Freshly ground white pepper

2 pounds soft tofu

1 cup crumbled goat cheese

2 large organic eggs, lightly beaten

½ cup freshly chopped flat-leaf parsley

1 teaspoon dried oregano

1 teaspoon freshly ground nutmeg

1 large onion, finely chopped

3 garlic cloves, finely chopped

3 cups Tomato Sauce (page 184)

Preheat the oven to 350 degrees F.

Place the eggplant on a nonstick baking dish and brush both sides with 3 tablespoons of the olive oil. Season with salt and pepper to taste. Bake 20 minutes or until tender but not brown. Remove from the oven and let cool.

Meanwhile, prepare the tofu mixture. Combine the tofu, goat cheese, eggs, parsley, oregano, nutmeg, and salt and pepper to taste in a food processor and pulse until well combined. Set aside.

In a large skillet, heat the remaining olive oil over medium heat. Add the onions and garlic and sauté until the onions are translucent, about 5 minutes. Add to the tofu mixture and combine thoroughly.

Ladle 1½ cups of the tomato sauce into a 9-by-13-inch baking dish.

After the eggplant has cooled, place a few tablespoons of the tofu mixture in the center of a slice. Gently roll the slice up and place it seam-side down in the baking dish. Repeat with the remaining slices until all of the mixture is used. Ladle the remaining tomato sauce on top.

Bake 35 to 40 minutes or until golden and bubbly. Remove from the oven and let cool a few minutes before serving.

Legumes and Whole Grains

Legumes are a low-fat source of complex carbohydrates, fiber, protein, and minerals such as potassium, magnesium, iron, copper, calcium, and zinc. Copper is responsible for strong collagen, which will keep your skin looking younger. Legumes include beans, peas, and lentils and are rich in the nutrients that your organs need to stay vibrant and in balance. They come in dried forms such as cannellini beans, adzuki beans, black beans, green split peas, and chickpeas, and fresh forms such as fava beans, string beans, cranberry beans, and sugar snap peas. It is suggested that some legumes help act as diuretics for your system, aiding the function of the kidneys, while others aid the function of the liver and pancreas. These organs need to be cleansed and nourished regularly with certain foods in order to stay strong and healthy. Eating legumes four to five times a week, along with a variety of herbs and vegetables, will result in clearer skin. Notice cultures that consume a lot of legumes in their diets. They age beautifully because their skin looks young and fresh.

Whole grains including quinoa, oatmeal (whole or rolled oats), bulgur, brown rice, wild rice, millet, spelt, amaranth, and kasha contain fiber, vitamins, minerals, and oftentimes protein. Some suggest that whole grains can help reduce your risk of heart disease and cancer. Whole-grain items can easily be incorporated into your diet, as they are usually quite easy to prepare and are good accompaniments to most entrées.

Fava Beans

Fresh fava beans are a springtime legume. Choose medium-sized pods, as they have a smaller seed and more delicate flavor. If the seeds are too big, you might want to peel them to make them more digestible. Fresh fava beans come in large, long (7- to 9-inch), thick pods with a white protective padding inside to protect the beans. Fava beans need to be shelled (removed from their pods). To open the pods, just pull on the stem at the top to unzip the string down either side of the pod, then gently push the pod open between your thumb and forefinger. Pop the beans out. If you are unable to find fresh fava beans, you may use frozen ones or lima beans instead. Frozen beans still have good nutritional value, since they are harvested at their peak season, then quickly frozen. Fava beans help act as a mild diuretic that can aid the body in reducing water retention and can also reduce puffiness around the eyes. • *Serves 4*

> 2 cups fresh fava beans *or* frozen baby lima beans, thawed
> 1 tablespoon extra-virgin olive oil
> 2 shallots, finely chopped
> 3 garlic cloves, chopped
> 1 teaspoon freshly chopped rosemary
> 3 tablespoons chopped Niçoise olives
> 1 cup Tomato Sauce (page 184)
> Sea salt
> Freshly ground white pepper

Bring a pot of water to a boil. Add the fava beans or lima beans and cook 10 minutes or until tender. Drain. Using the tip of a knife or your thumbnail, slit the translucent skin covering the fava bean, peel off, and discard. (If using lima beans, this is not applicable.) Set the beans aside.

In a large skillet, heat the olive oil over medium-low heat. Add the shallots. Cook 5 minutes. Add the garlic, rosemary, and olives and sauté 1 minute. Add the beans and tomato sauce and cook 20 minutes. Taste and add salt and pepper if desired before serving.

Lentilles du Puy

Like other legumes, lentils are low in fat and high in protein, fiber, minerals, and trace elements, and they have the added advantage of cooking quickly. Lentils have a mild, often earthy flavor, and they can be paired with almost any entrée. The best, most delicate lentils are the peppery French green lentils or lentilles du Puy. These hold their shape well but take a bit longer to cook than other lentils. They are good for the heart and the circulation, and increase the energy to the kidneys as well. Try serving salmon over a bed of these lentils. • ***Serves 4 to 6***

2 cups French lentils, picked over and washed in cold water
1 bay leaf
Sea salt
2 garlic cloves, thinly sliced
1 cup freshly chopped flat-leaf parsley
1 tablespoon extra-virgin olive oil
Freshly ground white pepper

Place 3 cups water, the lentils, bay leaf, salt to taste, and garlic in a pot and bring to a boil. Reduce the heat and simmer 20 minutes or until the beans are tender.

Drain the lentils and discard the bay leaf. Transfer to a serving bowl and toss with the parsley, olive oil, and salt and pepper to taste.

Chickpeas

Chickpeas or garbanzo beans are a good source of calcium, iron, and protein. They also contain a good amount of fiber, which helps cleanse the digestive system. • ***Serves 4 to 6***

> 2 cups dried chickpeas, soaked overnight in water to cover
> Sea salt
> 1 tablespoon extra-virgin olive oil
> 2 shallots, finely chopped
> 1 cup chopped Niçoise olives
> 3 garlic cloves, thinly sliced
> 1 cup Tomato Sauce (page 184)
> 1 teaspoon freshly ground cinnamon
> Freshly ground white pepper
> 1 cup freshly chopped flat-leaf parsley

Drain the chickpeas and rinse thoroughly. Place 4 cups water, the chickpeas, and salt to taste in a pot and bring to a boil. Reduce the heat and simmer 25 minutes or until the chickpeas are tender.

In a large skillet, heat the olive oil over medium heat. Add the shallots and sauté until tender, about 5 minutes. Add the olives and garlic and cook 1 minute. Add the tomato sauce, chickpeas, cinnamon, and salt and pepper to taste and cook 20 minutes. Stir frequently. Add a little water if needed to prevent scorching. Add the parsley and stir to combine. Taste and adjust seasonings if necessary before serving.

Soybeans

Native to East Asia, soybeans have been a major source of protein for more than five thousand years. Soybeans are high in protein (more than any other legume) and fiber, low in carbohydrates, and nutrient-dense. Compared with other legumes, soybeans are higher in essential fatty acids and are a good source of calcium, magnesium, lecithin, riboflavin, thiamine, fiber, folate (folic acid), and iron. All of these nutrients benefit your skin tremendously. • ***Serves 4 to 6***

1 tablespoon extra-virgin olive oil
1 small onion, finely chopped
1 stalk celery, finely chopped
2 garlic cloves, thinly sliced
2 cups frozen shelled soy beans, thawed
2 tablespoons Tomato Sauce (page 184)
2 bay leaves
Sea salt
Freshly ground white pepper
2 tablespoons freshly chopped flat-leaf parsley *or* tarragon

In a large heavy-bottomed skillet, heat the olive oil over medium heat. Add the onions and celery and cook about 5 minutes. Add the garlic and sauté 1 minute. Add the beans, tomato sauce, bay leaves, and salt and pepper to taste. Reduce the heat and simmer, covered, 30 minutes or until the beans are tender. Make sure that the flame is low enough so that the beans do not stick or get scorched. Before serving, add the parsley or tarragon and stir to combine. Taste and adjust seasonings if necessary.

Black Beans with Ginger and Cilantro

These delicious and flavorful beans are a good source of copper and other minerals, which help build collagen for smoother skin. • *Serves 4 to 6*

2 cups dried black beans, soaked overnight in water to cover

1 bay leaf

1 tablespoon toasted sesame oil

1 tablespoon freshly grated ginger

1 onion, finely chopped

1 carrot, finely chopped

2 teaspoons cumin

1 teaspoon turmeric

1 tablespoon garlic, finely chopped

Sea salt

Freshly ground white pepper

Juice and zest from 1 lime

2 tablespoons freshly chopped cilantro

Drain the beans and place in a large pot with cold water to cover and the bay leaf. Bring to a boil. Lower the heat to medium and cook 1 hour or until tender. Set aside.

In a large skillet, heat the sesame oil over medium heat. Add the ginger, onions, carrots, cumin, turmeric, garlic, and salt and pepper to taste. Cook about 5 minutes. Add the beans and stir until well combined. Cook 5 minutes. Just before serving, add the lime juice, lime zest, and cilantro. Taste and adjust seasonings if necessary.

Brown Rice Risotto

This recipe turns a classic northern Italian favorite into a fiber-filled dish that is great for your skin. Traditional risotto (often made with arborio rice) is prepared by slow cooking over low heat, adding liquid over time and letting it absorb to eventually reach a creamy consistency. This recipe uses the same technique but with a healthier grain. The result is a less creamy consistency with a strong, nutty flavor and chewier texture. Try adding some lightly cooked vegetables or grilled chicken or shrimp in the last few minutes of cooking for a heartier dish. • **Serves 4 to 6**

1 tablespoon extra-virgin olive oil

1 onion, finely chopped

2 cups short-grain brown rice

Juice and zest from 1 lemon

1 tablespoon freshly minced rosemary

1 tablespoon freshly minced thyme

Sea salt

Freshly ground white pepper

5 cups vegetable stock *or* chicken stock, heated to simmering

In a large skillet, heat the olive oil over medium heat. Add the onions and sauté until tender, about 5 minutes. Add the rice and stir until the rice is nicely coated with the olive oil. Add the lemon juice, rosemary, thyme, and salt and pepper to taste. Add the stock, one ladle at a time, stirring continually until each addition of stock is absorbed. Continue adding stock until the rice is tender but not mushy. Total cooking time should be about 45 minutes.

Remove from the heat, add the lemon zest, and stir to combine. Cover the rice and let sit for a few minutes before serving.

Wild Rice Salad

Wild rice is actually in the grass family and contains a lot of fiber. The ingredients in this healthy salad help reduce pore size, clear redness, and keep breakouts at bay for a clear complexion. Serve it with Wild Poached Salmon (page 143) or Herb-Roasted Chicken (page 130). • **Serves 4 to 6**

2 cups cooked wild rice

1 scallion, thinly sliced

1 teaspoon extra-virgin olive oil

1 carrot, finely chopped

1 stalk celery, finely chopped

½ cup finely chopped cherry tomatoes

1 tablespoon freshly chopped tarragon

2 to 3 tablespoons Lemon-Lime Olive Oil Dressing (page 177)

Sea salt

Freshly ground white pepper

In a large bowl, combine all of the ingredients and mix well. Refrigerate 1 hour before serving to enhance the flavor.

Quinoa Pilaf

This subtle, smoky supergrain is extremely rich in nutrients and contains up to 50 percent more protein than most other grains. Serve this tasty side dish with Pan-Roasted Monkfish with Miso Sauce (page 151) or Grilled Tofu (page 152). • **Serves 4 to 6**

> 2 cups quinoa
> 1 teaspoon extra-virgin olive oil
> 1 tablespoon minced garlic
> 1 tablespoon minced shallots
> ¼ teaspoon sea salt

Rinse the quinoa and drain through a fine sieve. Place the quinoa along with the remaining ingredients in a saucepan along with 3½ cups of cold water. Bring the contents of the pot to a boil. Cover and reduce the heat to a simmer. Cook 30 minutes or until tender. Drain excess water. Fluff and serve.

Millet Casserole with Tempeh and Arame Seaweed

Millet is a very alkaline grain. For my clients with rosacea, I suggest they eat it to help balance blood acidity, which I believe can cause rosacea. This dish will help to even out the complexion and remove reddening. Tempeh is a soybean-based low-fat protein with a nutty mushroom flavor. Seaweed's strong mineral content is beneficial for skin, hair, nails, and bones. Aside from tasting delicious, this casserole is rich in protein, minerals, and trace elements that help keep the body clean and well nourished. • *Serves 6 to 8*

4 tablespoons dried arame seaweed

1 tablespoon extra-virgin olive oil

8 ounces tempeh, cut into ½-inch cubes

1 large onion, finely chopped

1 carrot, diced

1 cup broccoli florets

2 tablespoons freshly grated ginger

3 garlic cloves, finely chopped

2 tablespoons toasted sesame oil

1 cup raw millet

2 cups vegetable stock *or* chicken stock *or* water

3 tablespoons tamari soy sauce

2 tablespoons toasted sesame seeds

½ cup freshly chopped cilantro

Sea salt

Freshly ground white pepper

Preheat the oven to 350 degrees F.

Soak the seaweed in cold water until it is tender, about 15 minutes. Drain and set aside.

(recipe continued on next page)

Preheat a nonstick skillet for 1 minute on medium-high heat. Add the olive oil. Place the tempeh in the skillet and sauté 2 to 3 minutes until golden. Transfer to a dish and set aside.

To the same skillet, add the onions, carrots, and seaweed. Sauté until tender, about 5 minutes. Add the broccoli and continue cooking for a few minutes until the broccoli is tender. Add the ginger and garlic and cook 1 minute. Transfer the tempeh back to the skillet. Remove from the heat and set aside.

In a separate skillet, add the sesame oil and millet. Let the millet "toast" for 2 minutes over medium heat, moving the pan constantly so that it does not burn. After 2 minutes you will smell a wonderful nutty aroma. When the millet starts to turn golden brown, add the stock or water and simmer, covered, 15 to 20 minutes.

Add the tempeh mixture, soy sauce, sesame seeds, cilantro, and salt and pepper to the skillet with the millet. Thoroughly combine and adjust the seasonings if necessary.

Place the mixture in a 9-by-9-inch oven-proof baking dish, cover, and bake 30 minutes. Remove the cover and brown the top under the broiler for 2 to 3 minutes. Serve immediately.

Vegetables

Vegetables are essential to our diet. They contain valuable vitamins, nutrients, and minerals that help fight disease. Try to eat a minimum of four servings of vegetables each day. Also try to consume a variety of red, yellow, and green vegetables daily to take advantage of the different beneficial elements they each contain.

Roasted Beets with Onions and Scallions

The minerals that are naturally contained in root vegetables such as beets help fortify the skin. This is a wonderful spring or autumn side dish that can be served warm or at room temperature. • *Serves 4 to 6*

2 pounds beets, cut into 1-inch cubes

1 large red onion, thinly sliced

1 bunch scallions, halved

1 tablespoon extra-virgin olive oil

1½ tablespoons red wine vinegar

Sea salt

Freshly ground white pepper

2 tablespoons freshly chopped flat-leaf parsley *or* basil *or* tarragon

Zest from 1 lemon

Preheat the oven to 375 degrees F.

Place the beets, onions, and scallions in a roasting pan and coat with the olive oil, red wine vinegar, and salt and pepper to taste. Roast 45 minutes or until fork tender.

Transfer to a serving bowl and sprinkle with the parsley or tarragon and lemon zest just before serving.

Mashed Celery Root

Root vegetables are beneficial for the skin because of the abundance of minerals they contain. The delicate, sweet flavor of celery root easily takes the place of mashed potatoes when you have the urge for something creamy. This is a good substitute for potatoes at Thanksgiving. Try serving with Roast Turkey (page 138). • **Serves 4 to 6**

1 teaspoon sea salt

2 pounds celery root, peeled and cut into small chunks

1 tablespoon extra-virgin olive oil

½ cup chicken stock

½ teaspoon freshly ground nutmeg

Freshly ground white pepper

Bring a pot of water to a boil. Add 1 teaspoon sea salt and and the celery root and cook 20 minutes or until tender.

Drain the celery root and puree in a food processor until smooth and creamy. Add the olive oil, chicken stock, nutmeg, and salt and pepper to taste. Mix thoroughly and serve.

Broccoli with Garlic

Broccoli is a cruciferous vegetable and is thought to help the body fight diseases including cancer. It has an abundance of vitamins, minerals, calcium, potassium, and fiber. You can prepare broccoli rabe and cauliflower the same way. • *Serves 4*

1 head broccoli, cut into florets
1 tablespoon extra-virgin olive oil
3 garlic cloves, thinly sliced
Sea salt
Freshly ground white pepper
¼ cup freshly chopped flat-leaf parsley *or* basil *or* tarragon

Bring a pot of water to a boil. Add the broccoli and cook 2 minutes. Drain the broccoli and quickly transfer to a bowl of ice water for a few minutes to lock in the color and stop the cooking process. Drain and set the broccoli aside.

In a large skillet, heat the olive oil and garlic over medium heat. Cook about 1 minute. Add the broccoli and salt and pepper to taste and sauté about 5 minutes. Add the parsley or tarragon just before serving.

Roasted Cauliflower

High in vitamin C, cauliflower is an excellent source of fiber, potassium, and nutrients that the skin needs to stay healthy and strong. Roasting vegetables brings out a natural caramelization, deep flavor, and crisp texture. Try preparing broccoli, brussels sprouts, or your favorite root vegetable the same way. • ***Serves 4***

1 head cauliflower, cut into florets
4 garlic cloves, thinly sliced
Sea salt
Fresh ground white pepper
1 tablespoon extra-virgin olive oil
½ cup freshly chopped flat-leaf parsley

Preheat the oven to 400 degrees F.

Bring a pot of water to a boil. Add the cauliflower and cook 1 minute. Drain and place in a baking dish. Add all of the remaining ingredients except the parsley, and toss until combined. Roast 20 minutes or until golden brown. Top with parsley and serve immediately.

Ginger-Steamed Baby Bok Choy

Bok choy has plump white stalks and deep green leaves. Part of the cabbage family, bok choy is rich in vitamin C and fiber. Bok choy is also a good source of folic acid. With its deep green leaves, bok choy has more beta-carotene than other cabbages, and it supplies considerably more calcium. The stalks and leaves have quite different textures, so it's like getting two vegetables for the price of one. I prefer baby bok choy because the leaves are more tender. Serve this with Asian Roasted Chicken (page 132) or Red Snapper with Shallot-Herb Sauce (page 144). • **Serves 4**

1-inch piece ginger, sliced

2 garlic cloves, sliced

1 teaspoon coriander

4 stalks baby bok choy, cut in half

1 tablespoon freshly chopped cilantro

Place 1 inch of water in a pot. Add the ginger, garlic, and coriander and bring to a boil. Carefully place a steamer basket in the pot. Add the bok choy to the basket and cook 2 minutes.

Transfer the bok choy to a serving platter. Sprinkle with cilantro and serve.

Sautéed Brussels Sprouts

Brussels sprouts help build your immune system by providing your body with disease-fighting nutrients. They are also high in fiber, which is great for your skin, as it helps to keep your system clean. Pan roasting the brussels spouts helps lend a sweet taste to the outer leaves, and pine nuts add a crunchy, nutty texture to the dish. • **Serves 6**

1 pound brussels sprouts, halved, outer leaves discarded
1 tablespoon extra-virgin olive oil
¼ teaspoon freshly ground nutmeg
Sea salt
Freshly ground white pepper
3 garlic cloves, thinly sliced
2 tablespoons toasted pine nuts
½ cup freshly chopped flat-leaf parsley

Bring a pot of water to a boil. Add the brussels sprouts and cook 4 to 5 minutes. Drain and set aside.

In a large skillet, heat the olive oil over medium heat. Add the brussels sprouts, nutmeg, and salt and pepper to taste and sauté until tender, about 5 minutes. Add the garlic and cook about 1 minute. Transfer to a serving dish and sprinkle with pine nuts and parsley just before serving.

Sautéed Red Cabbage and Apples

This dish is a wonderful accompaniment to roasted meats. It is perfect to serve in autumn when apples are at their peak season. • *Serves 4 to 6*

1 tablespoon extra-virgin olive oil
1 small head red cabbage, shredded
2 Granny Smith apples, peeled and thinly sliced
½ teaspoon ground cloves
½ teaspoon freshly ground cinnamon
Sea salt
Freshly ground white pepper

In a large skillet, heat the olive oil over medium heat. Add the cabbage, apples, cloves, cinnamon, and salt and pepper to taste. Cook about 20 minutes until everything is tender. Serve immediately.

Roasted Asparagus

Asparagus are a harbinger of spring. I eat them as often I can while they are in season. High-heat roasting helps bring out their flavor and adds a bit of natural caramelization. • **Serves 4**

1 1/2 pounds asparagus, trimmed
Juice and zest from 1 lemon
1 tablespoon extra-virgin olive oil
1/4 teaspoon freshly ground nutmeg (optional)
Sea salt
Freshly ground white pepper
1/4 cup freshly chopped flat-leaf parsley

Preheat the oven to 400 degrees F.

Place the asparagus in a baking dish and add the lemon juice, olive oil, nutmeg, and salt and pepper to taste. Toss until the asparagus are fully coated.

Bake 10 to 15 minutes. Sprinkle with the lemon zest and parsley before serving.

Dressings, Dips, Sauces, and Spreads

Here are some dressings, dips, sauces, and spreads that can enhance everything from salads to vegetables to fish to chicken. Try serving the dips and spreads with organic raw vegetables or toasted sprouted grain bread.

Lemon-Lime Olive Oil Dressing

Use this dressing the same day you make it to get the most out of the freshly squeezed citrus juice. Serve this dressing over salads, fish, and grilled chicken or tofu. • *Makes ¾ cup*

Juice and zest from 1 lemon
Juice and zest from 1 lime
4 tablespoons extra-virgin olive oil
¼ teaspoon sea salt
¼ teaspoon freshly ground white pepper

Whisk all of the ingredients together in a bowl and let sit 10 minutes before using.

Sherry Vinaigrette

This versatile dressing pairs well with almost any salad. I love it on Watercress Salad with Pine Nuts and Roasted Shallots (page 124) or on Beet and Goat Cheese Salad (page 125). Also try drizzling a little over grilled vegetables. • **Makes ¾ cup**

1 tablespoon finely minced shallots

2 tablespoons sherry vinegar

4 tablespoons extra-virgin olive oil

¼ teaspoon sea salt

¼ teaspoon freshly ground white pepper

Zest from 1 lemon

Whisk all of the ingredients together in a bowl and let sit 10 minutes before using.

Sesame-Ginger Carrot Dressing

This tangy Asian-inspired dressing is wonderful on Antioxidant Salad (page 122) or Wild Rice Salad (page 163). Also try serving it with grilled chicken or fish. • **Makes 1 cup**

2 teaspoons freshly minced ginger

2 garlic cloves, minced

2 tablespoons very finely chopped carrot

4 teaspoons rice wine vinegar

4 tablespoons toasted sesame oil

Juice and zest from 1 lime

2 teaspoons tamari or low-sodium soy sauce

¼ teaspoon sea salt

¼ teaspoon freshly ground white pepper

Whisk all of the ingredients together in a bowl and let sit 10 minutes before using.

White Bean Dip

I cut down on time when making this dip by using canned organic white beans. I serve this healthy and flavorful dip with raw vegetables when I entertain or spread it on a sandwich the next day. It will keep for up to 5 days in the refrigerator. • ***Makes 2 cups***

2 cups canned organic white beans, rinsed and drained
1 teaspoon freshly chopped rosemary
1 head roasted garlic (page 185)
2 tablespoons extra-virgin olive oil
Juice and zest from ½ lemon
Sea salt
Freshly ground white pepper

Place the beans, rosemary, garlic, olive oil, lemon juice, and lemon zest in a food processor or blender. Pulse until creamy. Add salt and pepper as desired before serving.

Hummus

This Middle Eastern dip is great with fresh vegetables or toasted sprouted grain bread triangles. Tahini is made from sesame seeds, which is an excellent source of antioxidants, vitamin E, and selenium to help fight free radicals and combat wrinkles. • **Makes 2 cups**

2 cups canned organic chickpeas, rinsed and drained
¼ cup tahini
Juice and zest from 1 lemon
½ head roasted garlic (page 185)
1 teaspoon cumin
Sea salt
Freshly ground white pepper

Place the chickpeas, tahini, lemon juice, lemon zest, garlic, and cumin in a food processor or blender. Pulse until creamy. Add salt and pepper as desired before serving.

Yogurt Herb Dip

This dip is great for the colon and digestion because of the natural acidophilus (healthy bacteria) found in yogurt. This versatile dip is also a good topping for grilled fish or chicken. • **Makes 2½ cups**

2 cups goat's milk yogurt
¼ cup freshly chopped flat-leaf parsley
¼ cup freshly chopped basil
1 tablespoon freshly chopped thyme
1 garlic clove, minced
Juice and zest from 1 lemon
Sea salt
Freshly ground white pepper

Combine all of the ingredients in a bowl. Chill 1 hour before serving.

Tzaziki

Made from thick, rich sheep's milk yogurt, this tangy Greek sauce is delicious served with vegetables such as eggplant and zucchini or as a dip for toasted sprouted grain bread triangles. You can also try substituting mint for dill. Cucumbers help hydrate the skin and fresh dill is great for cleaning out the system, resulting in a healthy, fresh complexion. • Makes 3 cups

4 Kirby cucumbers, finely chopped

1 teaspoon sea salt

1 quart sheep's milk yogurt, placed in a cheesecloth-lined
colander overnight to drain

½ cup freshly chopped dill

2 garlic cloves, minced

Juice and zest from 1 lemon

Sea salt

Freshly ground white pepper

Place the cucumbers in cheesecloth and sprinkle with the sea salt. Place the cheesecloth in a colander and allow the cucumber to drain for about 1 hour. Squeeze out any remaining liquid.

Place the cucumber in a bowl and add the remaining ingredients. Chill for a few hours if possible. Taste and adjust seasonings before serving.

Tomato Sauce

This basic tomato sauce is a staple in my kitchen. I mix it into soups, beans, and tofu dishes. It also goes nicely as an accompaniment to chicken or fish. • *Serves 4*

2 tablespoons extra-virgin olive oil
2 shallots, minced
3 garlic cloves, minced
1-pound can organic whole plum tomatoes, hand-crushed
6 freshly chopped basil leaves
¼ teaspoon freshly ground nutmeg
Sea salt
Freshly ground white pepper

Heat the olive oil over medium heat in a large skillet. Add the shallots and sauté 5 minutes. Add the garlic and cook 1 minute.

Add the tomatoes, half of the basil, nutmeg, and salt and pepper to taste. Cook 25 minutes over medium-low heat, stirring occasionally. Taste and adjust the seasonings if necessary. Add the remaining basil just before serving.

Roasted Garlic Spread

Some suggest that garlic can help boost your immune system and purify your blood, resulting in clearer skin. This rich, sweet roasted garlic can be used as a spread for sandwiches or to enhance the flavor of soups, roasted poultry, and vegetables. I always make extra to keep in the refrigerator. It will last up to 1 week. • **2 heads garlic**

2 heads garlic
¼ cup extra-virgin olive oil
1 tablespoon freshly chopped flat-leaf parsley
Sea salt
Freshly ground white pepper

Preheat the oven to 350 degrees F.

Cut the top quarter off each head of garlic. Please the garlic in aluminum foil and drizzle with the olive oil. Wrap the aluminum foil around the garlic and roast 45 minutes.

Remove the garlic from the oven and allow to cool. Squeeze all the garlic out of the skins into a small bowl. Add the parsley, salt, and pepper.

Juices, Smoothies, and Teas

Juicing is an inexpensive and highly beneficial way to create healthy, cleansing beverages. The cleaner your body is inside, the clearer your skin will be. Each 8 ounces of these delicious and refreshing homemade juices provides a boost of energizing vitamins, minerals, amino acids, enzymes, and nutrients that are quickly absorbed and delivered into your system. The best way to ensure that you are getting enough vegetables each day is to consume their beneficial elements in liquid form. As with everything else you prepare, I encourage you to use organic produce for juicing; otherwise, you may end up concentrating the pesticides from nonorganic produce.

Smoothies are a wonderful treat that the whole family can enjoy. For an extra protein boost, I like to blend in tofu.

Finally, as you know from the 7-Day Plan for Radiant Skin, I am a big fan of herbal teas for their calming and soothing properties. I've included a few blends for you to try.

Homemade Juices

These tasty juices are wonderful cleansers for your digestive system. Invest in a juicer and drink at least 8 ounces every day of this delicious energy boost.

Be sure to read the manufacturer's directions for your juicer before using. Choose any combination of fruits, vegetables, and herbs (limit herbs to a few tablespoons per 8-ounce serving) from the list below. Each juicer yields a different amount of juice, so you will have to experiment with quantities to get the amount you require.

apples	kale
basil	lemon
beet greens	lime
beets	papaya
blackberries	parsley
blueberries	pears
carrots	pineapple
celery	plums
cucumbers	strawberries
ginger	tarragon
grapes	

Green Apple Refresher

I recommend this bright green refreshing drink to clients who have problems with breakouts. It gently cleanses the system and helps keep pores clear of blemishes. • **Serves 1**

2 green apples, quartered
2 stalks celery, thinly sliced
Juice from ½ lemon
¼-inch piece ginger

Juice all ingredients according to the manufacturer's directions.

Pineapple-Basil Drink

This is a wonderfully refreshing fiber-filled beverage. I recommend it to my clients who are trying to control ruddy, oily complexions. • **Serves 1**

½ fresh pineapple, sliced to fit your juicer

2 tablespoons freshly chopped basil or tarragon

Juice all ingredients according to the manufacturer's directions.

Blueberry Smoothie

Start your day with this antioxidant-rich smoothie. Royal jelly is a resin produced by bees. It contains vitamins that are thought to benefit the skin. Aloe juice is extracted from aloe plants and is thought to have cleansing benefits. Slippery elm is an herb that may help gently cleanse and soothe the colon. All of these items are available at your local health food store or on-line. • **Serves 2**

1 cup blueberries

2 tablespoons royal jelly

½ cup aloe juice

2 cups unsweetened vanilla soy milk

1 teaspoon slippery elm liquid

1 teaspoon flaxseed oil

Combine all of the ingredients in a blender and pulse 1 minute. Drink immediately.

Strawberry Smoothie

This is a wonderful summer refresher. The tofu provides an added benefit of protein. Drink this for breakfast or during the day as a meal substitute for energy and maintenance. • **Serves 2**

1 cup strawberries
1 tablespoon royal jelly
3 cups unsweetened vanilla soy milk
1 teaspoon bran flakes
½ cup goat's milk yogurt
1 tablespoon ground flaxseeds
½ cup soft tofu
1 teaspoon flaxseed oil

Combine all of the ingredients in a blender and pulse until smooth. Drink immediately.

Papaya Smoothie

Papaya is one of my favorite fruits with its juicy, sweet-tart flavor and beautiful yellow-orange flesh. Some suggest that the enzymes in papaya are good for breaking down protein, which helps improve digestion. Papaya is a good source of vitamin C, vitamin A, and potassium. When buying papayas, choose those with a rich-colored skin that gives slightly to pressure. Slightly green papayas will ripen quickly at room temperature. • **Serves 2**

1 cup peeled, seeded, and chopped papaya
½ cup tofu
3 cups unsweetened vanilla soy milk
Freshly ground nutmeg to taste
1 teaspoon flaxseed oil
1 teaspoon ground flaxseeds

Combine all of the ingredients in a blender and pulse until smooth. Drink immediately.

Pineapple Smoothie

This tart, fresh, tropical smoothie is the perfect remedy for a hot summer day. Kids will love it, too. • **Serves 2**

1 cup chopped pineapple
½ cup tofu
3 cups unsweetened vanilla soy milk
1 teaspoon freshly grated ginger
3 mint leaves
1 teaspoon ground flaxseeds

Combine all of the ingredients in a blender and pulse until smooth. Drink immediately.

Ginger-Lemon-Chamomile Tea

I drink this soothing and refreshing tea at least once a day to help with digestion. I sometimes infuse rosemary and basil as well for their added health and beauty benefits. • **Serves 1**

1-inch piece ginger
½ lemon
1 chamomile tea bag
¼ teaspoon turmeric

Bring 2 cups of water to a boil. Steep the ginger, lemon, chamomile tea bag, and turmeric in water for a few minutes. Strain and serve.

Milk Thistle–Dandelion Tea

Milk thistle tea has a subtle taste and dandelion tea has a stronger, earthier quality. They are both available at your local health food store. I have used this tea as a natural diuretic to help cleanse my system for better skin. •
Serves 1

  1 milk thistle tea bag
  1 dandelion tea bag

Bring 2 cups of water to a boil. Steep the milk thistle and dandelion tea bags in the water for a few minutes. Serve.

FIVE

At-Home Spa Recipes
for Revitalized Skin

You feel it every day: the world whisking you off to another meeting, another school function, another stress-filled situation. The key is to find a haven where you can relax, regroup, and refuel. Creating an at-home minispa is that haven for escape. It's inexpensive, convenient, and the best way to practice the principles in this book. Meditation, exercise, relaxation, deep breathing, yoga, stretching, proper nourishment, and, of course, your new skin care regime are all things you can do at home. It may be hard to carve out time for yourself when you are a mother, spouse, executive, student, or all of these, but the good news is that there are treatments you can do at home to help you take care of your skin properly. For example, take an Algae Fine Powder Bath (page 49),

Epsom Salt Bath (page 48), or Apple Cider Vinegar Bath (page 48). Then apply your facial mask in the bathtub, which is the best place, since your skin is warm and your pores are open.

The following treatments should be done a minimum of once a week. Find the time to indulge in some soothing skin-care. The result will be radiant skin.

Herbal Skin Steaming

I recommend weekly steaming for all skin types, especially if you are suffering from a breakout. A good steaming with some common herbs such as rosemary and thyme will speed up the healing process. In the case of infectious breakouts (meaning those containing pus), eliminating red meat, cow's milk dairy, sugar, and junk food and replacing them with poultry, fish, fresh organic produce, nuts, and seeds can also help. Be sure to increase your dark, leafy green vegetable intake, too.

To prepare for steaming, wash your face with a fine gel cleanser and pat it dry with a clean towel. Always wash with warm water and rinse with cool so that you don't damage your capillaries.

Bring a medium-sized pot of filtered water to a boil. Add one sprig of rosemary or ¼ teaspoon lavender oil or 2 sprigs of thyme if you have breakouts. Adding 1 tablespoon of liquid golden seal and echinacea blend (available at health food stores) to the water helps boost the steam's antibacterial effect. If you have dry skin, add 2 bags of chamomile tea to the water rather than rosemary or thyme. Remove from the heat, cover the pot, and let it steep 5 minutes. Remove the lid and let the first steam escape so that you do not burn yourself. Drape a large towel over your head and carefully place your face over the pot so that the towel traps the steam. Make sure you are far enough from the steam so that it doesn't burn but close enough so that it feels warm and soothing. Steam your face for at least 2 minutes. Pull away from the pot for a few minutes. Then repeat until the water becomes lukewarm.

Balancing Facial Masks

After steaming, apply one of the following masks and leave it on at least 20 minutes. Rinse thoroughly with cool water and follow with your skin care routine.

Honey–Bee Pollen Mask

This mask that is designed for dry skin will rehydrate it and make it glow.

> 2 tablespoons raw organic honey
> 2 tablespoons crushed bee pollen

Combine the honey and bee pollen in a small bowl. Apply the mixture to a clean face and neck. Leave on 20 minutes. Rinse with cool water.

Oatmeal–Egg White Mask

This mask for oily skin helps remove excess oil and helps tighten and refine pores.

> 3 tablespoons oatmeal
> 1 egg white

Combine the oatmeal and egg white in a small bowl. Apply the mixture to a clean face and neck. Leave on 20 minutes. Rinse with cool water.

Oatmeal and Raw Honey Mask

Ideal for dry skin, this mask helps soften the skin, moisturizing the upper layers, leaving it vibrant and radiant.

> 1 cup oatmeal
> 1 cup filtered warm water
> ½ cup raw organic honey

Combine the oatmeal and warm water in a small bowl and allow the oatmeal to absorb the water. Add the honey and mix well. Apply the mixture to a clean face and neck. Leave on 30 minutes. Rinse with cool water.

Wheat Germ Mask

This mask is beneficial for normal to dry skin. It helps refine pores and make your skin soft.

3 tablespoons wheat germ
2 tablespoons warm water

Combine the wheat germ and warm water in a small bowl. Allow for the water to absorb the wheat germ. Apply the mixture to a clean face and neck. Leave on 20 minutes. Rinse with cool water.

Aloe and Cucumber Mask

This hydrating mask helps soothe irritated skin.

1 large aloe plant leaf, washed and chopped, *or* 1 cup aloe juice
1 cup chopped cucumber

Combine the aloe leaf (or aloe juice) and cucumber. Puree in a blender. Apply the mixture to a clean face and neck and leave on 30 minutes. Rinse with cool water.

Avocado and Lemon Juice Mask

Avocados are full of oils that help soften the skin and make it more radiant. Apply this mask weekly to dry skin.

    1 avocado, peeled, pitted, and mashed
    2 tablespoons raw organic honey
    2 tablespoons crushed bee pollen
    Dash of fresh lemon juice

Combine all of the ingredients in a food processor and puree. Apply the mixture to a clean face and neck. Leave on 30 minutes. Rinse with cool water.

Pineapple Pulp Mask

Whenever I juice pineapple, I drink one glass of juice, then take the pulp and put it all over my face and neck for a powerful natural peel that helps remove dead skin cells. Leave it on 20 minutes. Rinse with cool water.

Pureed Pumpkin and Prune Enzyme Peel

This peel is perfect for every kind of skin. The salicylic acid in pumpkin and prunes helps remove a buildup of oil in the pores and will brighten your complexion.

½ cup pitted prunes
½ cup canned pumpkin puree (not pumpkin pie filling)

Combine the prunes with 4 cups spring water in a pot and heat on low 30 minutes or until very tender and plump.

Combine the prunes and pumpkin puree in a food processor and pulse until a smooth paste forms. Apply the mixture to a clean face and neck and leave on 30 minutes. Rinse with cool water.

Essential Oil Premoisturizers

While using the right moisturizer on your face is important, it is just as beneficial to apply a premoisturizer. Choose the right premoisturizer for your particular skin type and apply it daily after cleansing and before your regular light moisturizer. Also apply a premoisturizer after using one of the balancing facial masks described previously. Be sure to use only a few drops at a time. Each batch of Essential Oil Premoisturizer should last a few weeks. For combination skin, apply Essential Oil Premoisturizer for Dry Skin around the periphery of the face, and Essential Oil Premoisturizer for Oily Skin around the T-zone daily.

Essential Oil Premoisturizer for Dry Skin

Combine 1 tablespoon macadamia nut oil, 1/4 teaspoon lavender oil, 1/4 teaspoon geranium oil, and 1/4 teaspoon basil oil in a clean glass jar with a lid. Shake well and gently pat a few drops onto your face, neck, and upper chest. Follow with an application of regular light moisturizer.

Essential Oil Premoisturizer for Oily Skin

Combine 1 tablespoon macadamia nut oil, 1/4 teaspoon lemon oil, 1/4 teaspoon lemongrass oil, and 1/4 teaspoon tea tree oil in a clean glass jar with a lid. Shake well and gently pat a few drops onto your face. (Always use the premoisturizer for dry skin on neck and chest.) Follow with an application of regular light moisturizer.

Essential Oil Premoisturizer for Sensitive Skin

Combine 1 tablespoon macadamia nut oil, 1/4 teaspoon camomile oil, 1/4 teaspoon rose oil, and 1/4 teaspoon rosewood oil in a clean glass jar with a lid. Shake well and gently pat a few drops onto your face, neck, and upper chest. Follow with an application of regular light moisturizer.

For the Body

While you may be concentrating on your face for ultimate skin care, don't forget about the rest of your skin and body! Here are two revitalizing treatments. I also recommend using jojoba oil combined with a few drops of an essential oil such as lavender oil or rose oil as a body moisturizer either on its own or under your regular body moisturizer for extra protection.

Salt Scrub

Use this invigorating exfoliation remedy from your neck to your toes!
Use a gel cleanser all over your body before using the scrub.

1½ cups kosher salt
1½ cups coarse Epsom salts
1 cup olive oil with 1 tablespoon scented oil such as lemon *or*
lavender *or* rosemary

Combine all of the ingredients in a bowl. Using your fingers, blend until the oil and salts are thoroughly combined. In the shower, use your hands and scrub your skin with the salt mixture beginning with your ankles and working up to the neck area. Pay close attention to the backs of heels, knees, and elbows. Rinse off well in the shower and finish with your favorite body lotion.

Deep Heat Rubbing Oil

I find this oil soothing for aching muscles. It also helps to relieve fatigue.

> **2 cups extra-virgin olive oil or canola oil**
> **1 teaspoon red pepper flakes**

Combine 1 cup of the olive oil and the red pepper flakes in a heavy-bottom pot and heat on low for 20 minutes. Strain the oil into a clean container and let it cool. Add 1 teaspoon of this hot pepper oil to the remaining cup of olive oil, mix well, and massage a small amount onto sore, tired muscles. Avoid getting the olive oil near your eyes or on your face. You can store the remaining hot pepper oil in the refrigerator for up to 1 month.

Skin Care for Men

While all of the information I've provided applies to both women and men, men require additional skin care because of daily shaving. As with women, I suggest men use gel cleansers instead of soap on their face and body. And like women, they should wash twice a day with warm water and rinse with cool water followed by application of a light moisturizer. Men should also perform a weekly at-home facial (page 52) for their skin type.

I recommend gel shaving creams rather than foam, as they tend to be less drying and irritating. For a better shave, place a warm, damp towel over your face for a few minutes before shaving. Apply the gel-based shaving cream and shave with upward strokes. If you suffer from razor burn, apply a solution of 1 teaspoon sea salt added to 8 ounces spring water after shaving. Apply as you would aftershave. Follow with a light moisturizer. If possible, try shaving every other day to avoid irritation. A few drops of vitamin E oil applied to the face and neck at bedtime will also help heal irritation caused by shaving.

Skin Care Through the Seasons

There are varying circumstances throughout the seasons that dictate what our skin requires to stay healthy, lush, and balanced. The environment plays a major role in keeping our skin balanced. Here are skin care suggestions for the demands presented by each season.

Spring

- Dry-brush your body (page 46) starting at the ankles and working your way up toward the heart to eliminate dead skin.

- Consult a yoga teacher to properly show you various poses that increase circulation throughout the body.

- Take revitalizing baths such as the Algae Fine Powder Bath (page 49) a few times a week for increased circulation, relaxation, and to alleviate muscle fatigue.

- Revitalize your body with a Salt Scrub (see page 204), which vigorously massages soothing mineral salts and oils into the skin to exfoliate and stimulate body circulation, leaving your skin smooth as silk.

- Stretch to increase circulation of the blood and lymph fluid. This relaxes your body, eases tension, and helps warm up and cool down muscles.

- Incorporate more fresh herbs into as many dishes as possible as they aid in digestion.

- Drink herbal or green teas, which are beneficial because of their cleansing and calming properties.

- Perform a 1-Day Super Cleanse once this season, where you consume only pineapple or papaya and water for an entire day. Both pineapple and papaya are high in enzymes that promote detoxification. The extra fiber will help cleanse your system and allow for more efficient elimination of toxins.

Summer

- Too much sun can cause skin damage including broken capillaries. Eating foods high in vitamin C such as berries, peaches, plums, kiwi, melons, broccoli, and kale can help build collagen.

- Keep sunscreen in your purse and apply a couple times a day. Use a minimum protection of SPF 15 every day, even on cloudy days.

- Increase your water intake by at least two glasses to compensate for sweating and to cool the body down.

- Avoid coffee and excessive alcohol because they dehydrate your body.

- Make sure that you are eating a variety of vegetables grown above the ground and below the ground to help your immune system stay strong.

- Perform a 1-Day Super Cleanse once this season, where you consume only pineapple or papaya and water for an entire day. Both pineapple and papaya are high in enzymes that promote detoxification. The extra fiber will help cleanse your system and allow for more efficient elimination of toxins.

Fall

- Exfoliate and peel dead skin naturally with a weekly Pineapple Pulp Mask (see page 200).

- It's cooler out and your body will naturally store fat to protect you from the cold. Limit your animal fat, but increase your intake of vegetable fats. Eat an avocado once a week and more nuts, seeds, and olive oil.

- Sprinkle an additional teaspoon of ground flaxseed on your cereal, favorite cooked vegetable, or salad. This will help bring out beauty and luster in your hair and skin.

- Perform a 1-Day Super Cleanse once this season, where you consume only pineapple or papaya and water for an entire day. Both pineapple and papaya are high in enzymes that promote detoxification. The extra fiber will help cleanse your system and allow for more efficient elimination of toxins.

Winter

- Increase consumption of vegetable fats, such as olive oil, nuts, and seeds, and fish fats, such as those found in salmon, mackerel, and sardines. Also try to eat more root vegetables such as yams, turnips, rutabagas, carrots, and parsnips.

- Eat an avocado once a week for the essential fatty acids it contains.

- Sprinkle an additional teaspoon of ground flaxseed on top of cereal, cooked vegetables, or salad. Flaxseeds also have essential fatty acids.

- Apply a weekly hydrating mask (pages 197–200) to your face to help prevent dry skin.

- Moisturize your body daily with jojoba oil, either under or over your daily body lotion, to help retain moisture.

- Reapply wrinkle cream or vitamin E oil frequently around your eyes and lips throughout the day to protect your skin from the elements.

- Use a cool-air humidifier to add moisture to the air. Make sure you clean it once a week or so, as it could harbor bacteria.

- Perform a 1-Day Super Cleanse once this season, where you consume only pineapple or papaya and water for an entire day. Both pineapple and papaya are high in enzymes that promote detoxification. The extra fiber will help cleanse your system and allow for more efficient elimination of toxins.

SIX

Healthy Body, Healthy Mind, Healthy Skin

A healthy body starts with a healthy mind. A healthy mind is created by clearing it of self-doubt, including thoughts such as I'm not good enough, pretty enough, rich enough, smart enough, and so on. Determine where the weak parts of your foundation are and strengthen each area physically, psychologically, and spiritually. The proper foods, yoga, meditation, and breathing exercises will all serve your life in a positive, healing way.

Just Breathe

According to Buddha, "You will not be punished for your anger, you will be punished by your anger." Whether it is anger, jealousy, family problems, fear, money issues, or just a busy and stressful lifestyle, negative and out-of-control emotions will punish your body and your skin. That's why it is essential to provide yourself with the tools necessary to put your life into a calm balance. Eating right and breathing properly are two of the most important tools.

Before you eat, take a look at your closed fist. Your stomach is about that size before you put food in it. Now look at the plate of food and the beverage in front of you, and remember the Eastern medicine guideline of one-third air, one-third food, and one-third water. Does the meal in front of you adhere to that balanced equation? It is far easier to adhere to this guideline if you eat small, frequent meals—up to five or six a day—rather than three large meals spread out over a 12- to 14-hour period. Proper digestion requires air or space in the stomach to move the food around and coat it with digestive enzymes. Also, frequent meals keep the metabolism working at a higher rate and more consistently.

Air, but more specifically, breathing, is essential for good health and efficient digestion. According to the National Institute of Aging, an active 45-year-old can be the biological equivalent of a 35-year-old, and an inactive 45-year-old can be the biological equivalent of someone aged 55. Breathing and breathing volume was found to play a huge role in the difference. As we inhale, oxygen comes into our system, purifies our blood, and removes waste through exhaling. But if breathing is irregular, shallow, or labored, the oxygen doesn't get a chance to do its job adequately. Subsequently, digestion may be interrupted and hindered, and our tissues, organs, and other systems may not get proper nutrients, making it nearly impossible for the body to function at its optimal level.

Next to eating right, breathing correctly is one of the best ways to keep the body running efficiently on several levels. On a physical level, proper breathing keeps the blood oxygenated, the mind and body relaxed, and the digestive tract functioning optimally. On a deeper level, however, breathing is essential to both psychological and emotional health. Breathing focuses the body and the mind, moving them into a rhythm that eases stress, lightens the spirit, and ultimately relaxes the body so that it can function properly. Eastern methods of healing and wellness have incorporated breathing exercises into their regimes for thousands of years, but only recently has Western medicine acknowledged their potential. Proper breathing can relieve anxiety, depression, indigestion, and any number of physical and mental ailments. And the best thing of all: learning to breathe correctly is simple, it takes very little time, physical or mental effort, and it's free!

Let's look at how you breathe now. If your chest or shoulders lift up when you breathe, if your breathing is short and quick or labored, you're not breathing correctly. To start, relax your mind with happy, pleasant thoughts. A friend once pointed out to me that because you can only think of one thing at a time, if you concentrate on good thoughts, you block out the bad ones. Keeping this in mind, inhale at a slow, even pace through your nose. Take an extra few seconds to exhale. This will let you absorb extra oxygen, remove carbon dioxide, and help you focus on something other than anxiety. Next, relax! Concentrate on your breathing from your diaphragm, a balloonlike pouch located under the lungs and rib cage. If you lie on your back, you will naturally breathe from the diaphragm. Put your hands on your abdomen. Breathe in and feel your abdomen expand and rise under your hands. Exhale and your abdomen will contract and drop back down.

Diaphragmatic breathing is the most effective form of breathing because it forces what experts have called maximum exhale. This will get rid of the most carbon dioxide from the lungs, which results in more room in your lungs when you inhale. The goal is to breathe this way while you're sitting or standing, which may take some practice. Take a deep breath at a comfortable pace, then at the top of the breath, release the air with a big, slow, even sigh. Try this a couple of times and feel the lightness your mind and body takes on.

Another one of my favorite breathing techniques for calming the whole body and mind is called Misogi, a Japanese technique used in preparation for engaging in martial arts. With Misogi, start by sitting upright and comfortably on your knees. This stimulates the energy in the stomach's meridian and is effective for assisting in proper digestion after you've eaten a meal. Inhale through your nose, then exhale through your mouth, making a "hahhhh" sound. Focus on your breathing and imagine it as a golden ring of light going in through your nose and out through your mouth. As with all breathing exercises, breathe diaphragmatically so that your abdomen expands and contracts.

Another breathing technique I like is based on Chinese medicine and the stimulation of the body's meridians, the pathways that help with digestion and circulation. This technique moves your nervous system from the fight-or-flight mode into the rest-and-digest mode. Put on comfortable, loose cotton clothes. Don't wear anything that is constricting or tight, especially around your waist. Sit in a straight-backed chair or on a meditation pillow up against a wall, and make sure you're sitting up straight but your body is comfortable. If you're sitting in a chair, make sure your feet are resting flat and comfortably on the floor, separated but relaxed. If you're on the meditation pillow, make sure your knees are bent but relaxed and your legs are flat on the floor. Relax your shoulders and your neck. Imagine a string pulling your head up so that it is straight but not rigid. Put your hands on your knees and make sure the heels of your hands are above the kneecaps and your fingers point downward.

With your index finger and thumb touching slightly, use your index, middle, and ring fingers to find the indentations in your knees below the kneecap. As you inhale, your breathing should gently expand your abdominal area. Don't force it. Let it happen naturally. As you exhale, you'll feel the abdomen contract and relax. Do this for at least 5 minutes after eating to get maximum benefit. And practice this breathing method if you experience minor indigestion.

Practice these breathing exercises upon waking, before retiring, or any time throughout the day. They are of great benefit to your body, mind, and skin.

Yoga and Digestion

Yoga is a six-thousand-year-old practice that combines a series of poses called asanas—breathing exercises and meditation to increase the body's health and physical, mental, and spiritual well-being. Yoga was conceived in India and made its way westward over the twentieth century to become the cornerstone of holistic health. Its benefits have even been touted by such mainstream organizations as the American Heart Association and Yale University's School of Medicine. Yoga can be credited with increasing energy and reducing blood pressure and body fat, but it is also valued for moving the body and the mind into a healthier, more relaxed state. When I was very young, I often found myself harboring a lot of stress. I would stretch to relieve the tension in my muscles and would instinctively assume what I found out later were yoga positions. These positions gave me the feeling of overwhelming energy and a sense of calm throughout my body. I have continued to study yoga ever since, incorporating it into my daily routine.

Eating on the run, being in fight-or-flight mode, and eating while agitated can wreak havoc on your stomach. If you don't digest your food properly, it cannot be assimilated into your system and waste cannot be eliminated. Yoga can help counter that. This chapter presents a 20-minute yoga practice that will assist the organs associated with digestion, assimilation, and elimination. The poses will also bring you peace of mind as energy flows through your system.

While making changes to achieve a healthier body, mind, and life, remember that it's a process. You probably won't achieve perfect yoga positions on the first try or even within the first week. That's okay! Each journey begins with one step and continues with another and another. Just keep in mind that this is a journey to health and beauty that is definitely worth the trip.

Be sure to consult your doctor before trying these yoga poses, as should be the case before beginning any new exercise program. Take your time and do as much or as little as you are comfortable with. Each day, week, or month, try and hold the pose for a bit longer, or keep trying to achieve a pose that may have been too difficult early on. Remember to always practice rhythmic breathing and be careful to not hold your breath.

Sun Salutation

What It Is

The Sun Salutation sequence helps you to move prana (energy) throughout your entire system by practicing a series of stretching and strengthening positions. This in turn helps digestion, elimination, and overall health and well-being.

How It's Done

The Sun Salutation starts with the body standing in prayer pose (Namaste). Stand tall with your eyes looking straight ahead of you, fixed on one point (about eye level on the wall), with your hands in prayer position in front of your heart.

Inhale a slow, deep, and long, gentle breath, bringing the air down to your pubic bone. Exhale slowly as you arch backward and find a point to look at on the wall behind you into a Backward Bend Pose.

Backward Bend Pose

What It Is

The Backward Bend Pose is beneficial to the digestive and eliminative organs in much the same way as the Cobra Pose. It increases the strength of the organs and directs the body's energy to digest and eliminate more efficiently, helping you get more nutritional value out of the food you're eating, while keeping your system cleaner by eliminating waste.

How It Helps Your Skin

The Backward Bend Pose increases efficiency in the digestion process and helps you achieve clearer, more radiant skin.

How It's Done

From a standing position, spread your feet about 1 foot apart with your hands either supporting your back or clasped together. Tuck in your pelvis to make sure that you bend evenly throughout your spine to distribute the arch equally up and down your back. As you are doing this exercise, focus not only on the motion but also your breathing. Inhale as you move into position.

Stay in the pose for 10 seconds, then slowly straighten back up to a standing and relaxed position while exhaling.

Standing Forward Bend

What It Is

After you perform a Backward Bend, you should do a Forward Bend to balance the body. So naturally the second part of the pose is a Forward Bend with the next exhalation.

How It Helps Your Skin

This pose focuses on the liver and kidneys to help improve digestion. It also stretches the lower part of the body including the hips, hamstrings, and calves while strengthening muscles in the thighs.

How It's Done

As you exhale, bend forward from the hips. If you can, keep your knees straight as you touch your hands to the floor. However, make sure you do not overextend your muscles. This is all a process, and you will achieve more and more flexibility as you practice. The purpose of this pose is to push your hips and buttocks upward while your hands and feet are pushing to the floor. If you can, put your hands next to either side of your feet with your fingertips facing forward. If you cannot bend that far yet, place your hands on your calves and hold the position there for 10 seconds as you gaze upward.

Put your hands on the ground and walk your feet backward until you end up on your stomach. From there, move into a Plank Pose.

Plank Pose

What It Is

The Plank Pose resembles the starting position for a push-up.

How It Helps Your Skin

It strengthens your upper body, especially your arms, while helping to strengthen your stomach and abdomen area. Abdominal strength is key to digestion, and digestion is key to clear skin.

How It's Done

From a prone position on your stomach, raise your torso up so that your arms are perpendicular to the floor, your back is straight, and you are balancing on your toes, similar to the beginning position of a push-up. Keep your body as parallel to the floor as possible with your head facing the floor. Try to hold the pose for 10 to 15 seconds.

Next, drop your torso onto the floor while lifting your head to stare straight ahead and keep your arms in an L with elbows on the floor and a slight arch in your back. This is the Cobra Pose.

Cobra Pose

What It Is

The Cobra Pose strengthens the spine, lungs, abdominal organs, and shoulders while assisting in digestion and elimination. In addition, it soothes many back problems by elongating and fortifying the muscles around the spine, opens up the respiratory and circulatory systems, and alleviates stress. It helps to clean out the kidneys and rid dark circles under the eyes. Breathing is very important with the Cobra Pose, as with any yoga pose or method of meditation. According to Yogajournal.com, the Cobra Pose also encourages the chest to open.

How It's Done

Start by lying on your stomach, legs straight back and flat on the floor. Place your hands under your shoulders with your elbows up against your body. Inhale and lift your chest off the floor, keeping your pelvis, legs, and feet flat on the floor. Tighten but don't tense your buttocks. Try to move your shoulder blades against your back and expand your ribs. Bend back as much as you comfortably can, but don't strain your back. Hold the pose for 15 to 30 seconds.

Downward-Facing Dog

What It Is

This position serves as both an overall stretch and a transitional pose.

How It Helps Your Skin

As part of a full-body routine, the Downward-Facing Dog energizes, aids digestion, stretches major muscle groups in the arms, legs, back, and spine, and strengthens the arms and legs.

How It's Done

From the Cobra Pose, push buttocks straight into the air to achieve the Downward-Facing Dog Pose. You will bend forward as you push up from the floor with both arms. At the same time, walk your feet toward your hands (with bent knees). Then straighten your legs so that your body becomes an upside down V with feet flat on the floor, arms extended in front of you, your head looking back between your legs. Keep trying to raise your hips and buttocks to the ceiling as you equally try to press the floor gently away from you. Hold that position for 10 to 15 seconds while breathing evenly before you move into the Upward-Facing Dog.

Upward-Facing Dog

What It Is

Similar to the Cobra position, the Upward-Facing Dog is an energizing stretch for the back, kidneys, and abdomen.

How It Helps Your Skin

Because this stretches and stimulates many of your internal organs including the stomach and lungs, it's enormously beneficial to the digestion process. It also strengthens the spine, buttocks, arms, and shoulders.

How It's Done

From the Downward Dog position, lower your body to the floor into the prone position with your legs straight back. Put your hands flat, palms down, fingers facing forward and spread on each side of your waist. Push up forward with your arms until they are straight and perpendicular to the floor. Your torso should be arched a few inches off the floor. The only thing touching the floor should be the palms of your hands and the top of your feet. Your head should be tilted toward the ceiling. Hold this position for 10 to 15 seconds, then release and relax onto the floor.

Bring the left leg forward with your knee bent and your hands on either side of your left foot, keeping your right leg straight back behind your body, as you look forward on the inhale, then bring your right leg to meet your left leg. In standing fetal position, try to touch your forehead to your knees, with your palms flat on the floor beside your feet and your fingertips facing forward. Hold this pose for 10 seconds, lovingly breathing into the back of your thighs, where you might feel a strain. This is normal in the beginning. Stand up straight on the exhale and go into a backward bend again. Finally, bring yourself into standing position with your hands in prayer pose, gazing at that same starting point on the wall in front of you.

Congratulations, you have just completed the Sun Salutation sequence or poses. Each time you perform this, it should be easier and easier.

Corpse Pose

After you have completed your poses, assume the Corpse Pose on your floor or mat to relax.

How It's Done

Lie on your back, legs out straight, hands at your sides, palms facing up. Relax and take a few deep, even breaths. Next, focus your attention on each part of your body, starting at the top of your head and moving slowly down to your toes. With each breath, relax your focal point, moving on to the next part of your body as is comfortable. At the conclusion of this exercise, remain in the Corpse position for 2 minutes. Then move into the Spinal Twist.

Spinal Twist

What It Is

The Spinal Twist gently strengthens and loosens the spine and nerves surrounding the spinal area. In essence, the movement associated with the Spinal Twist massages the liver, intestines, and spleen, encouraging smooth functioning and digestion.

How It Helps Your Skin

Because the Spinal Twist works on so many of the body's major organs, it keeps the assimilation and elimination processes working and the skin clear and toxin-free.

How It's Done

Start by sitting down with your legs extended on the mat. Turn your body to the right, with your right hand behind you. Make sure your right hand is close to but not quite touching your left buttock and that it is flat on the mat, with your fingers pointing away from your body. Follow by putting your left hand next to but not touching your right hand. Bend your left knee and cross your left foot over your right leg. Twist your head, neck, and body as far to the right as you can manage comfortably. Use your arms to balance and support you, but keep your buttocks flat on the mat and keep your spine as straight as possible. As you achieve the position, relax your back and try to look over your right shoulder.

Recommended Repetitions

Hold your breath and the position for 30 seconds (or as close to this as possible), then slowly exhale while you recenter yourself. Next, twist to the other side. After the Spinal Twist, repeat the Sun Salutation. Finish in the Corpse Pose.

In Closing

I hope *The Ciminelli Solution* has provided you with the tools to make healthy choices. Healthy skin is the result of a healthy body, healthy mind, and healthy lifestyle. Learning to let go of emotional pain, addictions, and unhealthy choices on a day-to-day basis is the cornerstone to achieving that healthy life. The more in touch you are with your inner self, the more you will be able see the cause and effect your past has on your present life. Each day is a new beginning. We're not perfect, but we can make better choices. Even following just a few of the suggestions in this book will result in changes to your body, mind, and skin that will impact and improve your overall health.

Make choices to put your health and wellness first. This is imperative not only to your survival but to your continued well-being, longevity, and ultimate beauty. Take time for yourself. Love yourself. Bring your body, mind, and spirit into balance to achieve lasting beauty. Your body is your temple. Treat it with love and respect.

I wish you a lifetime of good health and beauty.

SOURCES

Most of the items listed here are available at your local health food store as well as on these websites.

Acidophilus Probiotic
www.vitaminshoppe.com

Algae Fine Powder/Algae Deep Cleanse
www.susanciminelli.com

Aloe Juice (and other aloe products)
www.vitaminshoppe.com

Crushed Bee Pollen
www.vitaminshoppe.com

Essential Oils
www.florapathics.com

Crushed Flaxseeds
www.vitaminshoppe.com

Fruit and Vegetable Wash
www.shopnatural.com

Macadamia Nut Oil
www.botanical.com

Organic Produce and Poultry
www.diamondorganics.com

Royal Jelly
www.vitaminshoppe.com

Seaweed
www.asianfoodgrocer.com

Slippery Elm Liquid
www.vitaminshoppe.com

Smooth Move and Chamomile Teas
www.naturalwebstore.com

Vitamin E Oil
www.vitaminshoppe.com

To find out more about Susan Ciminelli products and services, visit www.susanciminelli.com. If you have a problem with your skin or have questions about what products you should use, e-mail Susan Ciminelli directly at asksusan@susanciminelli.com.

RECOMMENDED READING

I encourage you to read these books. The information they contain is compatible with the philosophies in *The Ciminelli Solution.*

Bieler, Dr. Henry G., *Food Is Your Best Medicine* (Bantam Books, 1987)

D'Adamo, Peter J., *Eat Right 4 Your Type: The Individualized Diet Solution to Staying Healthy, Living Longer & Acheiving Your Ideal Weight* (G. P. Putnam's Sons, 1996)

Hyman, Mark, *Ultraprevention: The 6-Week Plan That Will Make You Healthy for Life* (Atria, 2005)

Imus, Deirdre, *The Imus Ranch: Cooking for Kids and Cowboys* (Rodale Books, 2004)

Northrup, Christiane, *Women's Bodies, Women's Wisdom* (Bantam Books, 1998)

Northrup, Christiane, *The Wisdom of Menopause* (Bantam Books, 2003)

Pitchford, Paul, *Healing with Whole Foods: Asian Traditions and Modern Nutrition* (North Atlantic Books, 2002)

Rubin, Jordan, *The Maker's Diet: The 40 Day Health Experience That Will Change Your Life Forever* (Siloam Press, 2004)

INDEX

broccoli (*cont.*)
    in millet casserole with tempeh and
        arame seaweed, 165–66
brussels sprouts, sautéed, 173
Buddha, 212
butternut squash (roasted) soup, 119

carrot dressing, sesame-ginger, 179
cauliflower, roasted, 171
celery root, mashed, 169
cellulite, 9, 18–19, 46
chamomile-ginger-lemon tea, 192
chicken, 129–37
    Asian roasted, 132–33
    herb-roasted, 130–31
    okra stew, 136–37
    Tuscan, with rosemary and plum
        tomatoes, 134–35
chickpeas:
    basic, with tomato sauce, 159
    in hummus, 181
    and roasted garlic soup, 118
chicory, in cleansing salad, 123
cilantro:
    in adzuki bean soup, 112
    in Asian roasted chicken, 132–33
    black beans with ginger and, 161
    in chicken okra stew, 136–37
    in millet casserole with tempeh and
        arame seaweed, 165–66
    in seared sea scallops, 148–49
cleansing skin, 6–7, 43–44, 58
cobra pose, 221
collagen, 208
combination skin, 56–57
    7-day plan menus for, 61–79
Community Supported Agriculture
    (CSA) cooperative, 107
constipation, 1–2, 18–19
cooking at home, benefits of, 95–96, 109–10
corpse pose, 224
cosmeceuticals, 7
Crawford, Cindy, 7
cucumber(s):
    and aloe mask, 199
    in cleansing salad, 123
    in tzaziki, 183

dairy products:
    digestion and, 33–34
    healthy types of, 104
    skin care and, 4, 34
dandelion-milk thistle tea, 193
detoxification, 31–32
    basics of, 32–35, 38
    beverages for, 49–50
    daily skin care practices for, 58
    diet and, 32–37
    fasting and, 32–33
    of the kitchen, 97
    7-day plan for, 51–94
    skin care treatments for, 42–50
    tools for, 35–42
    yoga and, 40, 59
diaphragmatic breathing, 214
diet:
    detoxification and, 32–37
    dry skin type and, 52–53
    general health and, 8–9
    oily skin type and, 54
    seasonal skin care and, 207–10
    7-day plan menus and, 51–94
    skin care treatments and, 42–43
    skin health and, 4, 8–9, 26
digestion, 3, 110
    agitation and, 26–27, 59, 216
    breathing techniques and, 27,
        212–13
    dairy products and, 33–34
    improper nutrition and, 18–19
    skin breakouts and, 7, 18–19, 26–29,
        42–43
    yoga and, 216–17
digestive ailments, 26–29
dill, in tzaziki, 183
dips, 180–82
    hummus, 181
    white bean, 180
    yogurt herb, 182
"dis-ease" signs and signals, 20–23
downward-facing dog pose, 222
dressings, 176–79
    lemon-lime olive oil, 177
    sesame-ginger carrot, 179
    sherry vinaigrette, 178

dry skin, 52–53
    premoisturizer recipe for, 203
    7-day plan menus for, 61–79
dry skin brushing, 46
Dry Skin Essential Oil Premoisturizer, 53,
    56

eating small meals, 19, 212
eggplant tofu rollatini, 154–55
egg white–oatmeal mask, 198
Elizabeth (client), 22
endocrine system problems, 6, 28
environment and skin health, 12, 24–25,
    56
Epsom salt bath, 48
essential oil bath, 48
Essential Oil Premoisturizers, 44–45,
    53–55, 202–3
    recipes for, 203
exercise, 9
    aerobic, 32, 40–41
    detoxification and, 32, 40–41, 59
    yoga poses and digestion, 216–26
Ezekiel or sprouted grain bread, 100

facial masks, 3, 197–201
    aloe and cucumber, 199
    avocado and lemon juice, 200
    honey–bee pollen, 197
    oatmeal and raw honey, 198
    oatmeal–egg white, 198
    pineapple pulp, 200
    pureed pumpkin and prune enzyme
      peel, 201
    wheat germ, 199
fasting, 32–33
fats, "good" and "bad," 12–14, 34–35,
    108
fatty food intake, 27–28
fava beans, 157
fennel:
    in antioxidant salad, 122
    and red cabbage salad, 126
fiber intake, 33
fish and shellfish, 142–51
    Asian grilled tuna, 147
    lemon–rosemary grilled shrimp, 146

pan–roasted monkfish with miso sauce,
    151
    red snapper with shallot–herb sauce,
      144–45
    sautéed salmon with tomato and basil,
      142
    seared sea scallops, 148–49
    wild poached salmon, 143
    wild salmon burgers, 150
flaxseeds, benefits of, 102
flour, types of, 98
Food and Drug Administration,
    108
food shopping, 106–10
free radicals, 23–24
French lentils, in lentilles du Puy,
    158
fruits:
    cleaning, 36–37
    healthy types of, 104–5

garlic:
    in adzuki bean soup, 112–13
    in Asian roasted chicken, 132–33
    broccoli with, 170
    in chickpeas, 159
    in roasted cauliflower, 171
    in tofu casserole, 153
    in Tuscan bean soup, 114–15
    in Tuscan chicken with rosemary and
      plum tomatoes, 134–35
    in vegetable–stuffed turkey breast,
      140–41
garlic, roasted:
    and chickpea soup, 118
    in hummus, 181
    spread, 185
    in white bean dip, 180
gel cleansers, 6, 43
Gina (client), 14
ginger:
    in adzuki bean soup, 112–13
    in Asian grilled tuna, 147
    black beans with cilantro and, 161
    –lemon–chamomile tea, 192
    in millet casserole with tempeh and
      arame seaweed, 165–66

ginger (*cont.*)
    in pan-roasted monkfish with miso
        sauce, 151
    in seared sea scallops, 148–49
    -sesame carrot dressing, 179
    -steamed baby bok choy, 172
    in wild salmon burgers, 150
glycation, 14–15
glycolic acid treatments, 8–9, 53
goat cheese/feta:
    and beet salad, 125
    in eggplant rollatini, 154–55
    in fennel and red cabbage salad, 126
    in grilled zucchini and asparagus salad,
        128

Hall, Jerry, 5
herbal skin steaming, 45, 196–97
herb bundle, for wild poached salmon,
    143
herb-roasted chicken, 130–31
herbs and seasonings, fresh, 105–6
herbs and spices, dried, 98–99
herb yogurt dip, 182
Hoffman, Dustin, 7
holistic skin care treatment, 5
honey, raw, and oatmeal mask, 198
hummus, 181
hydrogenation process, 13, 108
"hypoallergenic" labels, 56

Iman, 5
immune system function, 20–21, 37, 42

Journal of Investigative Dermatology, 14
juices, 186–88
    green apple refresher, 187
    homemade, 186–87
    pineapple-basil, 188
junk food, 18, 59

kale:
    in creamy broccoli soup, 117
    in Tuscan bean soup, 114–15
    in vegetable-stuffed turkey breast,
        140–41
kitchen equipment, 96–97

labels on packaged foods, 108–10
Laura (client), 33–34
legumes, 156–61
    adzuki bean soup, 112–13
    black beans with ginger and cilantro,
        161
    chickpea and roasted garlic soup, 118
    chickpeas, basic, with tomato sauce,
        159
    fava beans, 157
    lentilles du Puy, 158
    mung bean vegetable soup, 116
    soybeans, 160
    Tuscan bean soup, 114–15
    varieties of, 99
    white bean dip, 180
lemon:
    in brown rice risotto, 162
    -ginger-chamomile tea, 192
    in grilled zucchini and asparagus salad,
        128
    juice and avocado mask, 200
    -lime olive oil dressing, 177
    in roasted asparagus, 175
    in roast turkey, 138–39
    -rosemary grilled shrimp, 146
    in Tuscan chicken with rosemary and
        plum tomatoes, 134–35
    in tzaziki, 183
    in vegetable-stuffed turkey breast,
        140–41
    in yogurt herb dip, 182
lentilles du Puy, 158
lime:
    in adzuki bean soup, 112–13
    in Asian grilled tuna, 147
    in Asian roasted chicken, 132–33
    in black beans with ginger and cilantro,
        161
    in chicken okra stew, 136–37
    -lemon olive oil dressing, 177
    in sesame-ginger carrot dressing,
        179

McDowell, Andie, 5
Macy's, 3
Maria (client), 24–25

massage therapy, 6, 22

men, skin care for, 206

menus for detoxification, 60–94

microdermabrasion, 8–9, 45

milk thistle-dandelion tea, 193

millet casserole with tempeh and arame seaweed, 165–66

Misogi breathing technique, 214

miso paste, 100

miso soup, 120

moisturizing skin, 44–45, 53

monkfish, pan-roasted, with miso sauce, 151

monosaturated fat, 13–14

mung bean vegetable soup, 116

National Institute of Aging, 212

"natural" foods, 109

normal skin, 52

    7-day plan menus for, 61–79

nuts:

    in fennel and red cabbage salad, 126

    types of, 102–3

oatmeal:

    -egg white mask, 198

    and raw honey mask, 198

oil, deep heat rubbing, 205

oils, types of cooking, 101

oily skin, 54–55

    premoisturizer recipe for, 203

    7-day plan menus for, 80–94

Oily Skin Essential Oil Premoisturizer, 54–56

okra chicken stew, 136–37

olives, Niçoise:

    in chickpeas, 159

    in fava beans, 157

    in tofu casserole, 153

onions:

    roasted beets with scallions and, 168

    in roast turkey, 138–39

    in Tuscan chicken with rosemary and plum tomatoes, 134–35

    types of, 101

organic produce, 9, 36–37, 59, 106–7, 109–10

Pacino, Al, 7

pantry staples, 98–106

papaya smoothie, 190

parsley:

    in antioxidant salad, 122

    in basic chickpeas with tomato sauce, 159

    in chickpea and roasted garlic soup, 118

    in creamy broccoli soup, 117

    in eggplant tofu rollatini, 154–55

    in herb-roasted chicken, 130–31

    in lentilles du Puy, 158

    in mung bean vegetable soup, 116

    in roasted cauliflower, 171

    in sautéed brussels sprouts, 173

    in tofu casserole, 153

    in Tuscan bean soup, 114–15

pesticides, avoidance of, 37

pineapple:

    -basil beverage, 188

    pulp mask, 200

    smoothie, 191

pine nuts:

    in sautéed brussels sprouts, 173

    watercress salad with roasted shallots and, 124

plank pose, 220

polyunsaturated fat, 13–14

premature aging, 8, 14–15, 17, 53

preservatives and additives, 16–17

processed foods, 2–3, 15–16, 34, 97, 109–10

product sources, 229–30

protein, healthy choices of, 106, 129

prune and pureed pumpkin enzyme peel, 201

pumpkin, pureed, and prune enzyme peel, 201

quinoa pilaf, 164

Rachael (client), 20

radicchio, in cleansing salad, 123

red cabbage:

    and fennel salad, 126

    sautéed, and apples, 174

red snapper with shallot-herb sauce, 144–45
reflexology, 2, 22
restaurants, healthy eating in, 110–11
rice:
    brown, in mung bean vegetable soup, 116
    brown, risotto, 162
    types of, 101
    wild, salad, 163
risotto, brown rice, 162
romaine lettuce, in antioxidant salad, 122
rosacea, 9, 17
rosemary:
    -lemon grilled shrimp, 146
    in roast turkey, 138–39
    Tuscan chicken with plum tomatoes and, 134–35
rubbing oil, deep heat, 205
Rubenstein, Helena, 7

saddlebags, 4, 9
salads, 121–28
    antioxidant, 122
    baby spinach and arugula, 127
    beet and goat cheese, 125
    cleansing, 123
    fennel and red cabbage, 126
    grilled zucchini and asparagus, 128
    watercress, with pine nuts and roasted shallots, 124
    wild rice, 163
salmon:
    sautéed, with tomato and basil, 142
    wild, burgers, 150
    wild poached, 143
salt intake, 15–16
salt scrub body treatment, 204
saturated fat, 13
sauces, 183–84
    miso, pan-roasted monkfish with, 151
    shallot-herb, red snapper with, 144–45
    tomato, 184
    tzaziki, 183
scallions:
    in Asian roasted chicken, 132–33
    in mung bean vegetable soup, 116

in pan-roasted monkfish with miso sauce, 151
    roasted beets with onions and, 168
scallops, seared sea, 148–49
seasonal produce, benefits of, 37, 107
seasonal skin care techniques, 207–10
seaweed, types of, 102
seeds and nuts, benefits of, 102–3
sensitive skin, 56–57
    premoisturizer recipe for, 203
Sensitive Skin Essential Oil Premoisturizer, 57
sesame, sesame oil:
    in Asian grilled tuna, 147
    in Asian roasted chicken, 132–33
    -ginger carrot dressing, 179
    in millet casserole with tempeh and arame seaweed, 165–66
    in miso soup, 120
    in pan-roasted monkfish with miso sauce, 151
    in seared sea scallops, 148–49
    in wild salmon burgers, 150
7-day treatment plan, 51–52
    for different skin types, 52–59
    healthy snacks for, 60
    menus and routines, 61–94
Seymour, Stephanie, 7
shallots:
    in Asian roasted chicken, 132–33
    -herb sauce, red snapper with, 144–45
    in roast turkey, 138–39
    watercress salad with pine nuts and roasted, 124
sherry vinaigrette, 178
shiatsu massage, 2
shopping for healthy foods, 106–10
shrimp, lemon-rosemary grilled, 146
silicone injections, 8
skin care:
    at-home spa recipes for, 195–210
    at-home tips for, 55
    avoiding soap and hot water, 6–7, 43–44, 58
    baths for, 47–50
    breakouts and, 7, 14, 18–19, 22, 26–29, 35, 42–43, 45, 196

breathing techniques and, 212–15
dairy products and, 4, 33–34, 104
detoxification and, 31–42
digestive ailments and, 26–29
"dis-ease" and, 20–23
distress signals and, 25–29
environmental factors and, 12, 24–25, 56
food recipes for improving, 110–93
free radicals and, 23–24
holistic treatments and, 5
improper treatments and, 7–8, 9
for men, 206
mental health and, 211, 213
proper cleansing and, 43–45
seasonal, 207–10
7-day treatment plan for, 51–94
stress reduction and, 1–2, 9, 22, 195–96, 212, 216
sun damage and, 24–25, 52–53
toxins and, 12–18
treatments, 42–50, 52–58
water intake and, 17–18, 20, 28–29, 33, 37–39, 52, 59
weight loss and, 14
skin care products, 5, 26, 53, 56
skin types, 57–58
    combination, 56
    dry, 52–53
    normal, 52
    oily, 54–55
    sensitive, 56–57
smoothies, 188–91
    blueberry, 188
    papaya, 190
    pineapple, 191
    strawberry, 189
snacks, healthy, 60
sodium nitrite, 17
soups, 111–20
    adzuki bean, 112–13
    chickpea and roasted garlic, 118
    creamy broccoli, 117
    miso, 120
    mung bean vegetable, 116
    roasted butternut squash, 119
    Tuscan bean, 114–15

soybeans, 160
spa recipes for at-home care, 195–210
    facial masks, 197–201
    herbal skin steaming, 196–97
spinach, baby, and arugula salad, 127
spinal twist pose, 225–26
spread, roasted garlic, 185
sprouted grain bread, 100
standing forward bend pose, 219
steaming pores, 45, 196–97
strawberry smoothie, 189
stress reduction, 1–2, 9, 22, 195–96, 212, 216
sugar:
    "disguised," 109
    types of, 14–15
sun damage, 24–25, 52–53
sun salutation pose, 217–18
Susan Ciminelli Spa, 8

teas, 192–93
    ginger-lemon-chamomile, 192
    milk thistle–dandelion, 193
teeth and tongue brushing, 41
tempeh, millet casserole with arame seaweed and, 165–66
tofu, 152–55
    casserole, 153
    eggplant, rollatini, 154–55
    grilled, 152
    in miso soup, 120
    in papaya smoothie, 190
    in pineapple smoothie, 191
    in strawberry smoothie, 189
tomato(es):
    in chicken okra stew, 136–37
    sauce, 184
    sautéed salmon with basil and, 142
    in tofu casserole, 153
    in Tuscan bean soup, 114–15
    Tuscan chicken with rosemary and, 134–35
    in wild rice salad, 163
toxins:
    alcohol, 17–18
    "dis-ease" and, 20–23
    elimination of, see detoxification

toxins (*cont.*)
    environmental factors and, 12
    free radicals, 23–24
    "good" and "bad" fats, 12–14, 34–35, 108
    immune system and, 20–21, 37, 42
    preservatives and additives, 16–17
    refined sugar, 14–15
    salt, 15–16
    white flour, 16
    trans fats, 13, 108
tuna, Asian grilled, 147
turkey, 138–41
    roast, 138–39
    vegetable-stuffed, breast, 140–41
Tuscan bean soup, 114–15
Tuscan chicken with rosemary and plum tomatoes, 134–35
tzaziki, 183

ulcers, 2–3
University of Maryland Medical Center, 13
upward-facing dog pose, 223–24

vegetable(s), 167–75
    broccoli with garlic, 170
    cleaning of, 36–37
    ginger-steamed baby bok choy, 172
    healthy types of, 104–5
    mashed celery root, 169
    mung bean, soup, 116
    roasted asparagus, 175
    roasted beets with onions and scallions, 168
    roasted cauliflower, 171
    sautéed brussels sprouts, 173
    sautéed red cabbage and apples, 174
   -stuffed turkey breast, 140–41
vinaigrette, sherry, 178
vinegars, types of, 103
Vitamin E oil, 45, 206

watercress salad with pine nuts and roasted shallots, 124

water intake, 17–18, 20, 28–29, 33, 37–39, 52, 59
Weaver, Sigourney, 7
weight loss, skin care and, 14
wheat germ mask, 199
white bean dip, 180
white flour, 16
whiteheads, 4, 33–34
white wine:
    in herb-roasted chicken, 130–31
    in sautéed salmon with tomato and basil, 142
    in vegetable-stuffed turkey breast, 140–41
whole grains, 156, 162–66
    brown rice risotto, 162
    millet casserole with tempeh and arame seaweed, 165–66
    quinoa pilaf, 164
    types of, 103–4
    wild rice salad, 163

Yale University School of Medicine, 40, 216
yoga, 2, 22
    detoxification and, 40, 59
    digestion and, 216–17
Yogajournal.com, 221
yoga positions, 217–26
    backward bend pose, 218
    cobra pose, 221
    corpse pose, 224
    downward-facing dog, 222
    plank pose, 220
    spinal twist, 225–26
    standing forward bend, 219
    sun salutation, 217–18
    upward-facing dog, 223–24
yogurt:
    herb dip, 182
    in strawberry smoothie, 189
    in tzaziki, 183

zucchini:
    grilled, and asparagus salad, 129
    in vegetable-stuffed turkey breast, 140–41